THE GREENWICH DIET

Lose Fat While Gaining New Health and Wellness

By Carlon M. Colker, M.D.

Medical Director, **Peak Wellness, Inc., Greenwich, CT**
Attending Physician, Medicine, **Greenwich Hospital, Greenwich, CT**
Attending Physician, Medicine, **Stamford Hospital, Stamford, CT**
Attending Physician, Medicine, **Beth Israel Medical Center, New York, NY**

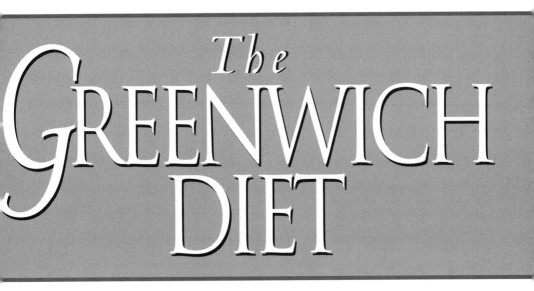

The GREENWICH DIET

Lose Fat

While Gaining

New Health

and Wellness

CARLON M. COLKER, M.D.

For information contact: Advanced Research Press, Inc.
150 Motor Pkwy., Suite 309, Hauppauge, New York 11788

The author has used science and experience to formulate the information presented in this work. However, this information is not intended to replace medical advice, as it is not the author's intention to offer diagnoses or prescriptions. Rather, the intent is to offer material that will help you, along with your physician, to develop the best, most appropriate health program for you to follow. Your physician should be consulted before you embark upon this, or any other, diet program; he/she is the best person to turn to for answers to questions or interpretations of symptoms. If you choose to use the information and programs outlined in this book without first receiving your doctor's approval, know that you are self-prescribing; the author and publishers assume no responsibility.

Individualization, according to physician guidance, is critically important to the success in any dietary, exercise or stress-reducing program, and such is the case with the Greenwich Diet. You know your own preferences and your physician knows your history. Together as a team, you are best equipped to determine the particular requirements that will meet your individual health needs and produce the best results.

Additionally, it would be a mistake to mix guidelines from this program with those of another program or plan without consulting your health care professional. Bring this book to your doctor. Once he/she has read and understood it, he/she can advise you. Always rely on your doctor's recommendations.

In particular, readers who have diabetes should be closely monitored by their physicians, as chromium may reduce the need for insulin. This program's ephedra-containing products are not designed for individuals with medical problems, including high blood pressure, heart disease, nervousness or anxiety. These products should also not be used by anyone taking a MAO inhibitor (an antidepressant), or anyone with the genetic disease PKU or existing pigmented malignant melanoma-type skin cancer. The products should be discontinued, until a medical professional has been consulted, if dizziness, sleeplessness, tremors, nervousness, headache, heart palpitations or tingling sensations occur. The diet program is not designed for women who are pregnant or nursing, or children under the age of 18, as the needs of these individuals are highly specialized.

All dialogue, quotes, statistics or anecdotes recounted in this text are actual and truthful, derived from extensive research and interviews. Nothing quoted has been printed without written permission. Any names used, other than those of the author, other authors, and scientific researchers, have been changed to ensure anonymity.

Library of Congress Cataloging-in-Publication Data
Carlon M. Colker, M.D.
The Greenwich Diet
1. Title
1. Diet   2. Low Carbohydrate   3. Nutrition
ISBN 1-889462-10-1

Printed in the United States of America

Jacket design by Thomas Tafuri
Illustrations by Lyman Dally

Dedicated to my parents, Edward and Elaine Colker, who gave me years of tutelage and guidance, and showed me limitless patience and understanding. Also, any lines on my face, they are from years of laughter. Thanks, guys.

ACKNOWLEDGEMENTS

To my immediate staff of unbridled enthusiasts—Melissa Swain, Douglas Kalman, Georgann Torina and Leonard Vigliatore for loving me unconditionally despite my near flawlessness and virtual lack of faults; (Relax guys! Where's your sense of humor.)

My assistant Alison Bologna, without whom I would be frozen like a deer in headlights at the daunting task of even attempting to organize my extreme existence without her.

My dear fellow workaholic colleagues Steve Blechman and Lauren Ruotolo for their fabulous input and thoughtful contribution to my work.

For guidance in the form of steadfast brilliance from Jon Whitcomb, as well as the inventive yet rugged genius of Paul Amadeo.

For inspiration from my sister Pamela (smooch), the strength and confidence of George Barasch (thanks for knowing me so well when it counted), a great friend and mentor Joe Weider, and sweet kindred spirits Roz and Jerry.

My patients, all of whom I am faithfully committed to.

In particular on this day, my star Greenwich Dieters George and Sonia who credit me with so much, but who perhaps do not realize how much more they give back to me with just their smiles.

To my many friends who power my senses and have meant so much to me, to name a few—Dominic N., Carlos S., Gary A., Dave G., Cathy K., Chris S., Jose A., Will B., Herb B., Vince B., Tony V., Jesse C., Channa C., Heather S., Rich D., Steve H., Rich C., Bill S., Paula D., E.D.D., Matthew L., Lynn G., Kelly H., Shara I., Mike J., Susan K., Chris K., Missy, and the entire Klug family, Matthew F., Shari L., Victoria L., Seth M., Scott M., Will V., Tom P., Todd P., Ronda S., Paula S., Illana Z., and so many more whom will not be forgotten;

And my bull, KZ, wherever life has taken him.

Contents

FOREWORD

As a cardiologist with a special interest in preventive medicine, I am particularly pleased to have the opportunity to introduce a significant new book authored by a colleague. In **The Greenwich Diet**, Dr. Carlon Colker has brought together several recent developments and concepts in the areas of clinical nutrition and metabolism and integrated them into a safe, clinically effective regimen usable by the typical individual wanting to lose weight.

Physicians are increasingly recognizing the impact of proper diet and nutrition on health and quality of life. It is now generally accepted that excess caloric intake, particularly in the form of carbohydrates, can result in the storage of excess energy in the form of increased body fat. But, we now know that even so-called "normal" carbohydrate intake can, and does, inhibit the burning of body fat for energy. This can result in the accumulation and retention of excess body fat.

The Greenwich Diet combines a reduced intake with an augmented protein allowance. It also incorporates fiber as an emphasized source for carbohydrate. Fiber is known to have the direct health benefits of reducing cholesterol and lowering blood sugar. It also promotes satiety, the subjective sensation of having one's hunger be truly satisfied by the portion or meal eaten.

The Greenwich Diet also incorporates whey as a major source of protein. Whey possesses one of the most complete amino acid profiles and highest biological value of any protein source, when compared to other available proteins, is significantly more bioavailable (assimilable in the diet). Within the diet's limited allowance of fat, there is an emphasis on the "healthy" fats. These fats, particularly the omega-3 and omega-9 fatty acids, are found in abundance in cold water fish and olive oil. They are known to lower blood fats and to improve the flow characteristics and clotting properties of the blood.

The Greenwich Diet has obvious similarities to the so-called "Heart Healthy Diet" that has recently gained acceptance by doctors, nutritionists and preventive health specialists. Its emphasis on low-saturated fat intake and on mono-saturated fats is also reminiscent of the "Mediterranean" diet that has been associated with enhanced heart health. It is a positive point that features of this diet draw from existing programs that were specifically designed for heart health.

The Greenwich Diet appears to be more balanced than the ultra low carbohydrate "quick fix" diets that claim to promote fat burning. This diet is user-friendly and can be followed as part of the healthy life-style of a reasonably motivated person. As a cardiologist, I have personally seen heart patients as well as motivated over-weight patients, comply with and benefit from following this novel program.

Robert M. Stark, M.D., FACC, FACP
Attending Physician, Internal Medicine & Cardiology,
Greenwich Hospital
a teaching affiliate of
Yale University School of Medicine

*I*NTRODUCTION

The last millennium is behind us. Looking back, we humans have had many accomplishments and made innumerable advances worthy of pride. Achievements in the arenas of science and technology, computers, engineering, communication and medicine are particularly awe inspiring. We have traveled into space and cured countless diseases. We have developed an interactive World Wide Web system of interconnecting people and places to communicate information. Our advances have made the world seem smaller, more manageable and more accessible than ever in history. Yet, despite our giant leaps forward, when it comes to the area of healthy eating for leanness, a disease-free body, energy and longevity, we have actually taken steps backward. Contradictory information, false promises, quick fixes, overstated claims, and poor real-life applicability have left people perplexed. But, believe it or not, through science and experience we have amassed enough knowledge—albeit fragmented—to figure out what's right. It is high time for a fusion of what we know. We must put a visionary approach to work in order to bring together our collective knowledge and produce a body fat-reducing, healthy-eating program for the new millennium. **The Greenwich Diet** is the product of just such an effort.

SHIFTING *the* PARADIGM

II

The Body in Transition

Breaking the Pattern

The reason the Greenwich Diet is so phenomenally successful is that it enlightens and empowers you through knowledge. This nutritional common sense elevates you far above the patterns of nonsense in which so many people are seemingly trapped. I liken this enlightenment to behavior modification.

Humans are not perfect creatures by any stretch of the imagination. In fact, we are terribly flawed in many ways. But who is to say we can't change? The only obstacle that holds us back is stubbornness and a lazy marriage to force of habit. The path to understanding the Greenwich Diet and reaching a new level of personal health and wellness involves battling patterns and tendencies toward "sameness" in order to make the seemingly unreachable suddenly achievable. Interestingly, this fight occurs only when one is resistant and close-minded. If one is willing to accept a new and better way of doing and being, the process becomes one of self-education.

Once you start implementing even a few simple principles of the Greenwich Diet you'll see how effortlessly you can shed excess pounds, feel better, and your commitment to these principles will grow exponentially. Eventually, you simply won't believe the almost childlike ease of it all. It will be hard to fathom how you ever got along without this basic knowledge.

People tend to be hopelessly caught in others' mind cycles of habits and opinions, so much so that it usually takes innovative thinking to break out of these stale paths to nowhere. But that means going against the grain. It means taking a chance and introducing a new idea or a new direction. Far too many people worship complacency and continue the walk through life in single file, heads down, never falling out of line and never looking for a different road.

Many current views on dieting and conventional "healthy" eating are examples of this pathetic cycle. Most people have absolutely no clue what they should be eating and what they should be avoiding. But once you learn the Greenwich Diet, you will have the knowledge that will last a lifetime.

The Principle of Starvation Alert

Apart from the different types of foods you should eat, one of the hallmarks of smart Greenwich Dieting is the temporal relationship of your meals. When you eat is as important as what you eat. In fact, you don't even need to eat very many calories at all, but if you eat them at the wrong time, you rapidly gain fat. It's a principle I call "starvation alert."

It's an age-old mechanism whereby your body attempts to resist change. Any warm-blooded animal has an internally programmed physiologic drive to preserve energy and not change when times are good. This is a condition called homeostasis, or literally, "pertaining to a condition of re-

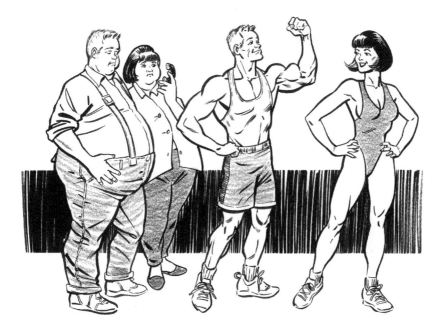

maining the same." When an African tiger, cheetah, or other predatory mammal has had unsuccessful hunts and has gone hungry for days, times are bad. The animal's body recognizes this, and internal adjustments are automatically made. The metabolism slows, hormone levels change and sleep patterns alter. The animals are in a state of starvation alert. But the moment they finally make a big kill and gorge themselves, their bodies exhibit an interesting response. They generally collapse and fall asleep from exhaustion even though they just ate massive quantities! This seemingly paradoxical response of their physiology actually makes a great deal of sense when you think about it. The period of starvation throws the body into a shocked state in which it makes necessary survival adjustments. These adjustments involve making fat storing pathways more energetically favorable. During such a state, even small amounts of calories can result in stored fat. This is the nature of the starvation alert mode—preparing for another imminent harsh time of deprivation by causing the body to hoard fat. At these times, the animals do tend to gain fat more readily to compensate for the period of starvation.

Sumo Wrestlers and Thanksgiving Day

My favorite example illustrating the principle of starvation alert in humans is the Japanese sumo wrestler. I have spent quite a bit of time in Japan and have made many close friends of Japanese heritage. As a result of my time spent abroad, I have come to know the Japanese culture fairly well. I can tell you that the Japanese are not an obese culture by any stretch of the imagination. In fact, traditionally the women are quite beautiful and lean, while the men are svelte and fairly fit. This is so much the case that it leads you to believe that genetics and not just dietary habits are at work here. But then, like a blip on a radar screen or a spike on a seismograph, emerging from these people of modest streamlined physiologic stature, is the sumo wrestler.

Thousands of years old, the sport of sumo seems more like a religious tradition at times than a sport. But these massive athletes are actually tremendously powerful wrestlers—albeit their power comes from fat! That's right, FAT. These men grow to staggering proportions, with some weighing well over 500 pounds. So, doesn't it make you wonder how a man from such an innately trim culture can produce so much fat? The answer is simple. It seems the Japanese have discovered the application of my theory of starvation alert and basically used it to create the otherwise inconceivable girth on these men.

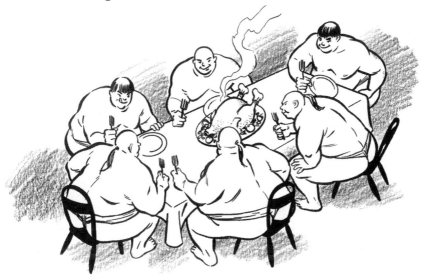

Contrary to what you might think, most sumo wrestlers traditionally eat only one meal a day, in the evening. It's called *chanko* and is made up of a pot of broth with pieces of meat, poultry, and fish mixed in with vegetables. The dish is served with a pot of rice and tea. It doesn't sound that excessive to most people and the majority of them are puzzled to figure out what is so bad about this meal. But, to the Greenwich Dieter, the problem is clear. Even though the total calories consumed are not that huge in number, the clear problem is one of timing. The meal is served in the evening and, worse yet, not long before going to sleep. The result is a cultivation of the worst aspects (for our purposes) of starvation alert.

Steeped in the tradition of sumo, they purposely starve themselves all day. This puts them into a state of starvation alert so that when the evening feeding comes, the body is fully prepared to hoard nearly every calorie as fat, all in preparation for what the body perceives as necessary for "surviving" the next period of deprivation. The other "rule" of gaining weight for Sumo is to have this single, isolated meal late in the day and then fall asleep immediately afterward. This again powers the hoarding of nearly every calorie as fat. Interestingly, as with animals, this extreme fatigue to the point of falling asleep is actually effortless, as it is an integral hallmark of a body being immersed in a deep state of starvation alert. Unlike the sumo diet, the Greenwich Diet simply does the reverse. Greenwich diet meals are smaller meals spread with frequency throughout the day with higher calories consumed in the morning, and decreasing throughout the day to nothing at bedtime. Once past the short adjustment phase, the Greenwich Diet allows your body to comfortably burn fat without pangs of hunger. Simply stated, in the same way sumo wrestlers have perfected the "art" of gaining fat, if you more or less reverse the model and do everything the opposite way in terms of meal patterns and timing, you've got the rhythm of the Greenwich Diet.

Perhaps the best common real-world example of my theory of starvation alert in action is Thanksgiving Day. It seems like everyone at one time or another has approached this gluttonous day with a similar flawed logic, and thus experienced the same outcome—starvation alert and subsequent fat gain. It starts a day or so before Thanksgiving. We begin holding back on eating in preparation for the large meal to come. Thanksgiving Day hits and we only have a cup of coffee for breakfast and skip lunch altogether, somehow thinking if we eat less during the day we will be able to get away with stuffing ourselves at night. Sound familiar? Just like the sumo wrestler, we have put ourselves in a state of starvation alert.

The subsequent result is that, in our deprived condition, we are primed to gain fat. We arrive at dinner famished. We gorge ourselves on turkey with gravy, stuffing, sweet potatoes, giblets and (let's not forget) cranberry sauce, among other yummies. What's the outcome? Well, if everyone else's diet theories about calories equaling energy were correct, we should be bouncing off the walls by now, right? In theory maybe, but in fact, quite the opposite happens. Like the predatory cat in the wild and not much different from the sumo wrestler, we are barely able to keep our eyes open. As we deliriously rise from the table with our belt buckles discretely undone, the blur of our gastronomically stretched consciousness comes into focus. Like fat lazy dogs, we eye a quiet warm spot on the carpet near the television and collapse into a deep sleep. That is, of course, until we come back to life about a half-hour later when someone wakes us up to ask us if we want some pumpkin pie!

DIETARY MISCONCEPTIONS and DISPELLING the MYTHS
III

The Great Carbohydrate Cajolery

One of the great dietary mistakes of the twentieth century is man's love affair with carbohydrates. It seems that everywhere you turn it's sugar, sugar and sugar. I don't speak just of simple carbohydrates like candies and fruits, but also of the complex sugars such as wheat products, rice and potatoes. In fact, as a clinician, I will venture to say that the terrible disease diabetes, which has plagued humanity in recent history, is more of a construct of man than an arbitrary malady that afflicts a victim without precipitation. In other words, we do it to ourselves. Feed the body the wrong substances and bad things will happen. I believe the same holds true for heart disease and cancer, but that link remains to be proven.

Here's the shocker—carbohydrate-based foods are simply unnecessary and harmful even in slight excess. When it comes to feeling good and looking good, relative to the other macronutrients like protein and fat, carbohydrates pale in comparison in terms of what they do to you. Protein, on the other hand, is absolutely essential. Without eating certain amino acids you will simply die because your body cannot produce them and must get them from the diet. Although some fats are harmful, certain fats are essential and must not be neglected in the diet. It is only the carbohydrates that have no essential character.

Our society fails to recognize the true lack of utility and actual inherent danger of an excess of carbohydrate-based foods. There are "low fat sections" in the grocery store that stock pastries and goodies with double the sugar of their full-fat counterparts. Labels brag about products that eliminate the fat, yet say nothing about excessive carbohydrate content. Sadly, the fat they have eliminated in some cases is the one true beneficial macronutrient in the product.

A Primordial Link

But it's not just society that is living this lie. Science also perpetuates the myth. To most scientists, carbohydrates equal energy. To "yours truly," also a researcher and physician, they simply don't. Fancy energy-producing metabolic cycles like anaerobic glycolysis or the aerobic Krebs cycle are showcased in textbook after textbook as carbohydrate dependent. But there are other pathways that feed these cycles quite efficiently and that originate from fat and even protein. The idea that carbohydrate metabolism is tightly linked to these cycles is a construct of man.

It was modern man who introduced carbohydrates into

the diet in great excess. Cave dwellers and early man foraged for food by killing animals and eating their meat, as well as gathering leaves, shrubbery and occasionally berries (all basics to the Greenwich Diet). They didn't boil potatoes, build rice paddies, harvest cornfields, or grind wheat. All these were developed much later by man to create filler in the diet and feed the masses.

The key to the Greenwich Diet lies in nurturing the primordial metabolic pathways back to life. These pathways, when stirred and challenged, are actually extremely efficient energy producers. By retraining your metabolism, you will shed your dependence on carbohydrates.

Bears Don't Bake Biscuits

The same lessons can be learned from the animal kingdom. For example, bears don't bake biscuits! Like humans, bears are mammalian omnivores (i.e., eating both meat and vegetables). In the wild, bears grow to majestic heights and are heavily muscled. They are powerful and athletic animals that if provoked can close 50 yards on a man in seconds. They eat foods like salmon, rabbits, rodents and other small animals, as well as an enormous amount of leafy greens, nuts and berries. In the zoo, it's a different story. Despite massive developments built for them, they always look docile and sluggish. They mope around and sleep a lot. In fact, bears in captivity don't even hibernate as they do in the wild, but still look fat all year-round. So, what's the problem with these furry fellows? You guessed it—carbohydrates. It seems many of the larger zoos have taken to feeding the bears enormous amounts of "bear biscuits." So, what the heck is a bear biscuit? Fortunately, my research staff was

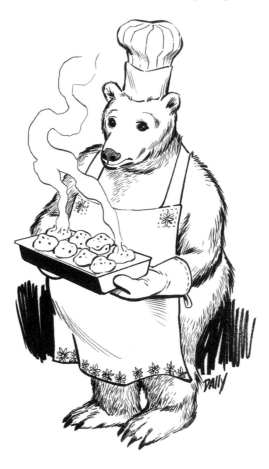

aggressive enough to find out and contact the company that makes them. Simply put, it is a cornmeal-based nutrient biscuit. Can you believe it? As if it isn't bad enough that man has diverged so far from the nutrients needed for healthy living, we have sunk to victimizing the bear with our flawed paradigm. Oh, the "bear-manity"!

Popular Protein Distortions

Protein—Not Guilty by Association

Unlike fat, which has been directly targeted for complete avoidance in many diets, protein was not directly targeted as much as it was a casualty of fat avoidance behavior. Traditionally, people have avoided what they consider to be fatty foods and in the process eliminated red meat, eggs, milk and poultry from their diets. It is my steadfast belief that protein deficiency, which is rampant in society, especially among women, is a result of a systematic and proactive elimination of some of the healthiest foods known to mankind.

The Fat-Burning Power of Dietary Protein

Metabolism can be affected by the foods you eat, as well as other things. Some raise your metabolism (i.e., certain supplements or medications), while others slow the metabolism (i.e., yo-yo dieting, etc.). One of the keys to long-term weight control is understanding how foods can affect your metabolism. Protein has a natural metabolic advantage, and thus is a cornerstone of the Greenwich Diet.

The process of the body burning food for energy is known as the thermic effect of food (TEF). The TEF varies for each macronutrient. That is, the thermic effect of protein, carbohydrates and fats varies individually. Since most people eat mixed meals, the total TEF is usually an average of these components. The combined TEF of protein, carbohydrates and fats together elevates basal metabolism by usually no more than 10 percent. This is due to the high amounts of carbohydrates and saturated fats most people usually eat in a meal. Individually, each macronutrient is assigned a TEF value. Of these, ingestion of both carbohydrates and fats elevate the metabolism by only five percent, while protein ingestion elevates basal metabolism by up to 25 percent. Clearly, there is a protein advantage.

Supporting this idea that protein actually boosts metabolism is a study demonstrating that meals containing 68 percent protein, compared to either 68 percent carbohydrate or fat, resulted in subjects consuming more protein to burn 66 percent more calories. This simple principle of protein having TEF superiority is utilized by Greenwich Dieters to control weight.

Protein Causing Renal Failure? Nonsense!

The claim that an excess of dietary protein somehow causes renal failure in healthy adults is perhaps the most annoying and outlandish piece of diet misinformation repeated throughout the media and popular press. This belief is not just a simple media distortion, but also rather a colossal fabrication that has even made its way into nutrition textbooks. As a result, many of my highly respected physician colleagues continue to espouse this nonsense.

The start of this misconception began with early observations of protein intake in patients with kidney failure. What was noted was that an excessive amount of dietary protein in the form of meat, fish, milk and eggs, seemed to gradually worsen the functioning of their kidneys. Of course, this is a logical conclusion in these individuals because the kidneys are quintessential in the final excretory process of amino acids (the building blocks of protein). As a result, the idea that excessive dietary protein can worsen kidney function has obtained widespread acceptance. But remember that this observation was only in individuals with a disease or illness that had abnormally affected their kidneys. Nonetheless, this has somehow come to mean that protein is in some way going to harm healthy adults with no kidney problems.

An example to illustrate how ridiculous this misinterpretation is, would be to take individuals with "bad" hearts (i.e., congestive heart failure with decreased ventricular function) and rigorously run them around an indoor track. Although mild exercise is recommended for most of these patients, exercising at this level of intensity for these types of people will likely result in a heart attack and/or death for many. Does that mean running around a track will cause a heart attack and death for a normal, healthy adult? Nonsense! Get my point? In fact, for a normal, healthy adult it's quite the contrary. Running around a track is not only indicated but also extremely healthy.

Sadly, this misconception has pervaded popular thinking about protein. Yet, nothing could be further from the truth. The position of the National Kidney Foundation, which seems to be continually ignored by naïve physicians and dietitians, is clear. The Foundation does not have, nor has it ever had, a position on protein as a cause of kidney disease or on any relationship of protein to kidney disease in the healthy adult.

Beyond our own American foundation, consider the report published in the *European Journal of Clinical Nutrition*. It clearly states there is no obvious upper limit of protein intake that healthy adults cannot accommodate to. In fact, it goes on to discuss strength training athletes taking in four grams per kilogram per day of protein and experimental studies where subjects were given as much as eight grams per kilogram per day of protein without any harm to the kidneys.

Recall my example of early man and what constituted his diet. This primordial link is what we have deviated far from as a society. In fact, it is estimated that Paleolithic diets were more than half protein. As an interesting aside, men in the famous Lewis and Clark expedition across America ate as much as nine pounds of buffalo meat each day with no ill effects. That's well over 600 grams of protein as a daily minimum! In today's world, although too low in fiber consumption, only the Eskimos and gauchos of the Pampas predominantly consume protein in the form of fish and meat, respectively. They are not exactly Greenwich Dieters, but I can assure you they don't have kidney failure as a result of the protein they eat.

Soy Protein

For years we have thought soy and soy proteins are healthful. Mass cultivation of the soybean for food started as early as 1500 B.C. in Asia and continues to enjoy great popularity.

Although the soybean is the most complete of the vegetable proteins, it is still debatable among scientists and nutritionists as to whether or not soy is a complete protein. Again, unlike meat proteins, vegetable proteins usually lack a relatively large number of the essential amino acids (those building blocks of protein we cannot synthesize in the body and thus must ingest in our food). Soy protein, although unusually complete, may lack one or more of the essential amino acids (in particular, methionine). In fact, it is because of this debatable completeness that many sports nutritionists shy away from recommending soy protein to athletes.

If we focus on the lack of methionine in particular, which we know is missing from soy, the inferiority compared to other animal source proteins quickly reveals itself. Methionine is an unusual and valuable essential amino acid in that it contains sulfur, thus making it a very important amino acid for tissue growth and development (anabolism). In addition, because of its sulfur component, this particular amino acid is needed for proper immune function by helping to increase concentrations of the powerful intracellular antioxidant known as glutathione (GSH). Think carefully about these reasons because they are at the crux of the reason why the soy over-enthusiasts call this "just" a conditionally essential amino acid. (By the way, many textbooks don't buy into this logic either, and simply list methionine as an essential amino acid.) I guess it is true you can survive on soy as long as you are not physically challenged and never fall ill. But it won't work if you need that little extra help a protein rich in methionine could provide. For active, healthy wellness-oriented folks following the Greenwich Diet, lacking a conditionally essential amino acid is as bad as lacking an essential amino acid.

Further, although soy may in fact promote health in certain women because of its phytoestrogen (estrogen-like) properties, the same quality may also seriously disturb healthy hormonal balance in others. This may seem shocking to some and, although theoretical, it must be considered. The phytoestrogen in soy that has received so much press is a subcategory of an isoflavone called "genistein." As a potent antioxidant, it is believed genistein may be able to block key enzymes that tumor cells (cancer) need to grow. Early research with genistein has shown some efficacy in shrinking tumors, although not uniformly. Most scientists consider the research on genistein inconclusive, while the media has had a ball with it. Nonetheless, despite the media favorite this little word has become, it is far from the world's panacea.

Keep in mind that as a health choice for certain carefully screened individuals, soy does seem to lower cholesterol.

Also, in certain women, soy seems to help relieve some of the symptoms of early menopause, as well as slow bone loss in perimenopausal women, thus possibly preventing osteoporosis. These are all fine qualities, but remember, that doesn't make soy a good protein. Instead, it only says that soy is a good "medicinal food" for certain individuals. Sadly, the press and even scientists seem to get this confused. They can't seem to understand that, even though soy may offer these benefits in certain people, it should never be eaten at the cost of true protein. If it is taken as an adjunct to healthy complete protein and you are properly screened to demonstrate that you have a likelihood of benefiting from soy, I have no objection to it occupying a place in the diet in small amounts. But again, for the reasons outlined, soy doesn't count as a protein in my book.

Fat Falsity

Good Fat, Bad Fat

For what seems like forever, we've been fed false propaganda that "fat is bad." We've been told to avoid fat in the diet at all costs. This is not only a theme in magazines and tabloids, but it also emanates from scientific literature.

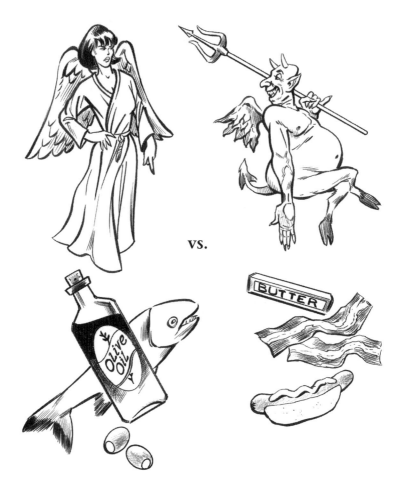

vs.

Unfortunately, especially in the case of scientific literature that we rely upon as heavily factual, this information couldn't be further from the truth. The truth is that, like protein and unlike carbohydrates, fat is essential. In other words, without the proper fat in your diet, you will die.

All of this "fat is bad" propaganda probably stemmed from early calorie counting. One gram of either protein or carbohydrate is equal to four calories, while one gram of fat equals nine calories. Per gram, fat has more than double the calories of protein or carbohydrate foods. It seems that this single comparison has woefully distorted the facts. This archaic perspective takes none of the many good qualities of proper fat into account. In fact, our knowledge has evolved considerably since the early days and we are just now realizing how absolutely vital proper fats are in the diet.

Why would your body store something if it didn't have an exceedingly efficient way to access the storage? Was God just asleep on the job? When it came to figuring out why we have fat, was he just having a bad day? I mean, think about it. Would you ever put something in storage with no easy way to access it if you needed it? Of course you wouldn't. In fact, sanity dictates that people store things in places they can get to. It makes sense. Yet incredibly flawed logic has prevailed in America and the wheels of propaganda have supported the avoidance of fat. But the truth is your body can easily access body fat and efficiently use it for energy if you train your body to do so with the Greenwich Diet.

Modern man has basically substituted carbohydrates for fat with the misperception that carbohydrates equal energy. Unfortunately carbohydrates do nothing but keep you fat. After all, why should your body learn to burn off the layers of fat and use stored fat as energy when you are pumping in a steady flow of sugars? Simply stated, your body will take the path of least resistance until it is conditioned otherwise. This reconditioning of the metabolism is what we do with the Greenwich Diet. We recondition your body to reacclimatize itself to efficiently and preferentially use fat for energy.

In fact, it is amazing to see the paradoxical response experienced when seasoned Greenwich Dieters reintroduce carbohydrates into their system. It is almost as if their bodies don't know what to do with this unhealthy sugar and, rather than sugar giving them "energy" as most over-weight people claim, it actually fatigues the Greenwich Dieter. Many even report falling asleep! So, we can retrain our bodies to recapture the essence of how we were meant to function. It's heartening to watch my clients tap into fat burning efficiency and shed their fat at a rate they never thought possible while picking up boundless energy.

Clamoring About Ketosis

Ketosis is a state characterized by an accumulation of substances in the blood called "ketones" (specifically, ace-toacetate, beta-hydroxybutyrate and acetone). The presence of ketones in the blood is signified by a "spilling over" of ketones in the urine. These ketones can be easily detect-ed. Ketosis actually signifies a condition whereby the body relies on stored body fat to provide energy to the brain, organs and tissues. Not a bad thing at all when you think about it. So, why has it received such widespread negative press? Well, classically, in the medical and scientific literature, ketosis has always been considered to be of concern because the condition was traditionally associated with starvation. Other pathologic conditions associated with ketosis have included uncontrolled diabetes mellitus and inadequate nourishment during pregnancy. So, with all the fearful associations, it comes as no surprise that ketosis has received such a bum rap. But I posit that the bad propaganda surrounding ketosis is more distortion than fact.

Commonly, high-protein, low-carbohydrate diets are considered ketogenic because they can cause ketosis. During a prolonged fast, the body's carbohydrate stores are quickly depleted, resulting in lower levels of blood glucose. Although it's classically considered critical to maintain a certain blood sugar level to provide the brain with energy, if the transition to lowering carbohydrates is gradual enough, the body then uses fat and protein for energy. In order to preserve protein, the body uses less glucose and relies more strongly on fat metabolism. Sounds logical, right? However, fat is unable to cross the blood-brain barrier and provide energy to the brain. As a result, the liver converts these fats to ketones, which the brain readily uses for energy.

The body has a very efficient and sensible metabolic pathway involving ketones. Just because the formation of ketones results from some abnormal and/or disease conditions, this hardly means they have anything to do with causing such conditions (a fact many people ignore). Ketones are not some kind of nasty byproduct of toxic destruction. They actually have great usefulness. When our bodies are tuned and centered, we awaken metabolic pathways that have long been forsaken. When we stop the narcotic diet of overfeeding our bodies carbohydrates, we rediscover old energy routes of great efficiency that don't require ingesting sugar foods for energy.

As long as you experience only a mild, transient ketosis and you are sure to include adequate amounts of essential vitamins, minerals, and fiber from vegetables, you are probably on the right track. Of course, severe ketosis can result in nausea, hypotension, dehydration and fatigue. But these are usually only seen in cases associated with starvation. In the absence of severe dehydration and metabolic stress, starvation ketosis does not normally progress to ketoacidosis, a condition in which the plasma ketone concentration becomes high enough to cause a dangerous drop in pH (i.e., the blood becomes more acidic). In fact, there is little evidence in the literature to suggest that ketogenic diets actually induce ketoacidosis. This is largely due to the fact that dietary protein, if high enough, can be converted to carbohydrates. In fact, a study from the Department of Nutritional Sciences at the University of California-Berkeley showed that a hundred grams of dietary protein provides about 55 grams of carbohydrates, which is more than enough to prevent ketosis. Thus, if liberal amounts of protein are regularly ingested, ketosis should not be an issue.

Because of this lean away from carbohydrates, the Greenwich Diet might be classified by some as a mildly ketogenic diet. However, such a label is incorrect. Actually, the Greenwich Diet is high in protein and has incidental carbohydrates (from vegetables), essential fats, fiber, water, and other essential nutrients, thus making ketosis unlikely and infrequent except during the more focused fat-burning stages. This allows the pathway of mild transient ketosis to actually work for you, rapidly but safely stripping the body of flab during times of more intensified dieting.

$\mathcal{M}$ACRONUTRIENTS & NUTRIENT CATEGORIES
One-By-One

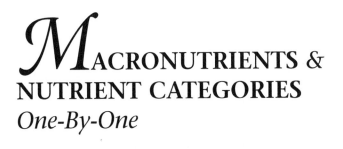

Carbohydrates

A Background on Carbohydrates

Carbohydrates are sugars. As such, they have traditionally been viewed as the fuel for most body functions. In fact, glucose (the simplest single molecular form of sugar) marks the beginning of the energy-utilizing pathway known as glycolysis. This method is anaerobic and yields ATP (the true currency of energy in the human body). At the terminal pathway of glycolysis and under aerobic conditions, glucose ultimately becomes pyruvate and with the help of various enzymes, enters the Krebs cycle.

Both the glycolytic and Krebs cycles have been exhaustively studied because simple organisms have had to rely heavily on these cycles to create a more efficient utilization of energy and subsequently evolve. Of course, since these cycles begin with a molecule of glucose, it should come as no surprise that carbohydrates have literally become the star of the show in terms of the traditional scientific and textbook definitions of our dietary source of energy.

I would remind my medical and scientific colleagues that what might be true for microorganisms and lower life forms along our evolutionary path, has little bearing on higher organ function, as in humans. What I'm saying is that, although carbohydrates have always been thought to be the major fuel source of human energy, this could not be further from the truth. Carbohydrates have become so important because we as a society have made them so. By stoking our furnaces with an excessive amount of dietary carbohydrates, we have in essence created a lazy path of least resistance. This sugar-coated trail allows our bodies to get away with ignoring the very efficient metabolic routes of fat burning for energy and protein utilization when necessary.

In an effort to dispel this carbohydrate myth, re-education of the public must take place. Let's take a step back and look at carbohydrates from a more conventional standpoint. Different types of carbohydrates are valued differently. There are both simple carbohydrates (sugars) and complex carbohydrates (starches).

As mentioned, glucose is the simplest of all carbohydrates and exists as a single molecule. However, the public generally doesn't consume pure unprocessed glucose. Instead, the classic example of simple carbohydrate form that pervades the American diet is "sucrose" in the form of table sugar. Thus, any type of candy, including cookies, cakes, pies, ice cream, and the like are loaded with sugar. Interestingly, although natural, fruit juices and most fruits (especially dried) also contain a significant amount of simple carbohydrate, in the form of fructose and not table sugar.

The problem with these simple carbohydrates is that they fall into a category we call "high glycemic index" foods. As such, they are absorbed quickly into the bloodstream and cause a rapid increase, or "spike," in blood glucose and insulin levels. Repetitive insulin spiking as a result of a persistently elevated blood sugar causes insulin resistance, which explains the high incidence of diabetes in our society. In addition, insulin can switch on a body fat-producing metabolic pathway called "lipogenesis." This, of course, easily explains the pervasive obesity in our society and it should be easy to see how sugar—in the form of high-carbohydrate foods—is basically killing us.

Perhaps the biggest current bamboozling taking place is on our grocery store shelves. Since dietary fat is equated with body fat, coupled with the fact that one gram of carbohydrates is equal to four calories while one gram of fat is equal to nine calories, carbohydrates have come to be perceived as "good" while fat has been labeled "bad." Pastry companies have wasted no time in exploiting this distorted propaganda to generate profits. In so doing, "fat-free" cakes and "cholesterol free" cookies have popped up everywhere. Playing on the guilt of the public, these products fly off the shelves and into the mouths of plump consumers who have the notion that somehow they are doing some good for themselves. The problem is that simple carbohydrates in particular, although lower gram for gram in calories than fat, are far more calorie dense. In other words, although a product might be "fat-free," in truth the product may be so densely loaded with carbohydrates that the calorie equivalent is the same, or even more! Add to that what we know about the insulin spike caused by simple sugars. Although not a fan of fatty foods (the Greenwich Diet tends to avoid animal fat with exception of fish oils), given the choice, I actually would prefer a moderate amount of fat over a blast of simple carbohydrates.

Carbohydrates can also be complex. Glucose may be strung together in strands to form polysaccharides, otherwise known as complex carbohydrates. They may also be in the form of starches, such as pasta. Complex carbohydrates are more filling and give you lower intensity levels of energy yield, but over longer periods of time. Complex carbohydrates are digested and broken down more slowly. As a result, the absorption is also slower. In sharp contrast, simple carbohydrates need little digestive processing and are thus absorbed quickly, explaining insulin spiking.

So, clearly carbohydrates of the complex type are more favorable. However, Greenwich Dieters take it one step further and limit the type of complex carbohydrates to those that are fiber based. In fact, the fiber element is so important in the Greenwich Diet that the carbohydrate-containing foods are almost strictly vegetables. The carbohydrates in them are what I call "incidental." In other words, they are foods that are low in carbohydrates but high in fiber. For example, even though corn is a vegetable that is relatively high in fiber, it is more of a complex carbohydrate in the form of a starch. Thus, it is not a regular part of the Greenwich Diet. On the other hand, veggies like broccoli, cauliflower, cabbage, lettuce, celery, spinach, peppers, zucchini, squash, carrots, onions and cucumber are all healthy choices.

I believe our society has been sickened by an overabundance of carbohydrates in the diet. For example, diabetes is considered one of the most common diseases known to man, yet I believe we, as a society, have made it so. If we didn't pump our children and ourselves with carbohydrates from day one, most people with diabetes would live a normal life having never known or suffered from the condition. It's the sugar that brings it out. As a society, we have fooled ourselves into thinking that carbohydrates are synonymous with energy. In a healthy body, nothing could be further from the truth. We even ignore our own science, which tells us that changes in amino acid oxidation lead to alterations in the pathways used to produce energy. This happens in such a way that if protein is high enough, the utilization of protein for energy becomes the favorable pathway. Excess proteins, in the form of amino acids, are oxidized in the body and easily contribute nearly 60 percent of the energy we need. Most of the remaining energy needs come from fat, with only a small portion from carbohydrates. This only occurs in a healthy body with a well-primed metabolism, and that is what you achieve on the Greenwich Diet.

Five Basic Carbohydrate Rules of the Greenwich Diet

1. 30-100 grams of carbohydrates for non-exercisers, 50-200 grams of carbohydrates for exercisers. If you are used to taking in a lot of carbohydrates, work this level down gradually and pay attention to your body because too drastic a drop is unnecessarily uncomfortable, not to mention, unmanageable.

2. With the exception of what might be contained in one of your dietary supplements, you should be consuming incidental carbohydrates only. (Your only source of sugar should be from the carbohydrates that happen to occur in relatively small amounts within fibrous vegetables). Ingest no carbohydrate-based foods.

3. No starchy foods (rice, pasta, white bread, potatoes, corn, etc.). Learn the difference between a carbohydrate-based vegetable like corn or yams and a fiber-based vegetable like broccoli or spinach. Although bread is not part of the Greenwich Diet, if you are tempted on rare occasion, a heavy whole-grain bread in moderation and in the morning or mid-afternoon isn't such a terrible thing.

4. Avoid fruits. Don't kid yourself; they are simple sugars. If you feel you need one once in a while, choose apples because of their relatively high fiber and pectin content.

5. At least in the beginning, while building up your fiber intake, be sure to take a good daily multivitamin/multimineral supplement so your body isn't missing any of these elements.

Protein

The Story on Protein

As we age, our protein levels drop significantly. Total body protein levels in healthy older adults are only about 70 percent of those found in young adults. This suggests an urgent need for dietary protein. Protein intake is directly related to energy intake and although people tend to decrease their caloric intake as they age, protein intake remains considerably higher than the RDA (recommended dietary allowance). Protein deficiency is much more common than we physicians would like to believe. A protein deficiency not only destroys the immunity of a person, it leads to a myriad of other problems. In short, a deficiency in protein is a prime accelerator of illness, fat gain and the aging process.

Next to water, protein is the most common substance in the body. And because of the versatile properties and malleable nature of protein, it has an infinite number of applications. As a nutrient, proteins have many different functions and are part of every cell in the body. Your body requires a constant supply of protein to repair cells as they wear out and are replaced by new ones. During times of growth, such as infancy, childhood, adolescence and even pregnancy, the body needs extra protein to make new body tissue. In addition, proteins regulate body processes. As enzymes and hormones, proteins make various chemical reactions occur. As antibodies, they help protect the body from infection and disease.

Proteins are fundamental, integral and essential food components. They are the source of amino acids, which are essential for growth, tissue repair and DNA/RNA synthesis. Providing the foundation for everything from enzymes, to hormones, to cells, proteins make up the framework of an infinite number of compounds and structures in the body. Protein has many applications as a "functional food" because of its unique properties. Commercially available proteins are obtained from animal or plant sources. The proteins obtained from animal sources and used as food ingredients include gelatin, egg products, milk and fish. Leaves, stems and roots have been explored as possible sources of protein, with the seed being the most useful part of a plant. Although incredibly poor quality, wheat and corn have also been used as protein sources in bakery and breakfast foods. The proteins you are most likely to be familiar with are non-fat dry milk powder, egg protein, egg white powder, casein and whey.

Proteins are made up of a combination of approximately 20 different amino acids. Like fats and carbohydrates, the amino acids that make up any protein are composed of carbon, oxygen and hydrogen atoms. However, proteins contain nitrogen, which makes their structure and role in health unique. Of all the amino acids, only about nine are "essential." Commonly listed essential amino acids include histidine, isoleucine, leucine, lysine, methionone, phenylalanine, threonine, tryptophan, and valine. These amino acids are deemed essential because they are not manufactured by the body from other substances and hence must be obtained from food.

Certain proteins are known as "complete" proteins because they contain all the essential amino acids. They are pretty easy to remember since nearly every type of animal meat is a complete protein and thus contains all the essential amino acids. Examples include beef, milk, poultry, eggs and fish.

Unfortunately, commercially available proteins are obtained from a variety of sources, both animal and plant. The complete proteins obtained from animal sources and used as food supplement ingredients include eggs, egg products, milk, milk products and meat. Some are better sources than others, but all of these are complete.

Conversely, there are "incomplete proteins." These proteins are deemed incomplete because they lack one or more of the essential amino acids. Vegetable source proteins are examples. Leaves, stems and roots have all been found to be incomplete. Wheat and corn are also incomplete non-animal source proteins.

The key point to understand is that complete protein is absolutely necessary in maintaining health, promoting proper bodily function, supporting immunity, keeping youth intact, and preserving wellness. What is important is that animal source protein be an integral part of your daily diet. (Don't think God gave you incisor teeth for no reason—they're for tearing flesh, not just shrubbery). But keep in mind, it's the new millennium and the latest food technology is all around us. If eating meat turns you off, that's okay. You can still get the complete protein your body needs from supplementation.

Whey is the Way

Given all that we know about protein, it should be evident that not all proteins are created equal. *Whey protein lacks no essential amino acids in any form. As a result, it has a much higher biological value in terms of similarity to our own human protein.*

Skim milk is the starting point for the manufacture of a host of milk products. Milk contains two major proteins, casein and whey. Casein is actually the principal protein of milk. The manufacture of casein involves an extraction process and can be obtained by the acid treatment of whey itself. Casein is said to have a biological value (BV) of 77, which means that your body may only absorb 77 percent of the available protein. In contrast, the biological value score of whey is 104. Hence, when comparing casein with whey, whey wins out.

The fact is, whey protein has the absolute highest biological value of any available protein (i.e., *BV* Whey— 104, *BV* Whole Eggs—100, *BV* Egg White—88, *BV* Casein— 77, *BV* Soy—74). Whey proteins are found in meal replacement powders, enteral solutions and reduced fat products. Whey protein is rich in branch chain amino acids, cysteine, lactose, minerals, lactalbumin and traces of fat. Standard processing removes microbes and other impurities, thus allowing for a purer product. This is something for those individuals with lactose intolerance to keep in mind because the filtration processes allow for the removal of lactose in some forms of whey supplements (i.e., whey protein isolates): In this case, whey protein can be considered more "consumer friendly" when compared to proteins like milk or eggs to which so many people are intolerant or even allergic.

Whey protein is a by-product of cheese manufacturing. Recent scientific research on whey has produced impressive results. Rich in the branched chain amino acids, whey protein, with its high biological value, is perhaps the perfect energy source for the muscles of a dieting and exercising individual. Whey protein has been shown in many studies to help protect the body from oxidative stress, viral infections and cancers by enhancing the immune system.

We have all heard of vitamins E and C and their antioxidant ability in the bloodstream. However, a far more powerful and target-specific antioxidant exists within each living cell called L-gamma-L-glutamyl-L-cysteinyl-glycine (sorry, folks). We just abbreviate this rather clumsy name as "GHS." This powerful antioxidant exists and exerts its action within the cell. GSH is an essential antioxidant that protects cells and serves as a primary detoxifier of harmful substances that attach to our cells' DNA. Insufficient GSH levels have been associated with diseases such as AIDS, heart disease, Alzheimer's and Parkinson's disease.

The problem is that GSH can only be synthesized inside the cell from smaller molecules. This is because there are no efficient transport mechanisms in the body to get GSH from the blood stream into the cells. Basically, all we can do to be sure we have enough GSH within our cells is provide the "bricks and mortar" to transport into the cells for assembly into GSH. Look at it like trying to set up a large bed frame in your bedroom. You can't move it all in at once, it simply won't fit. But, if you bring it in piece-by-piece and then assemble it, there's no problem.

With this model in mind, the key building block for GSH is an amino acid called cysteine. When two molecules of cysteine are coupled together and linked by a disulfide bond, the result is a molecule called cystine. This cystine molecule is not only stable, but travels easily through the body and into each living cell. Once in the cell, it is broken down into cysteine molecules and used to form the powerful antioxidant GSH.

Unlike proteins such as soy, whey protein (in particular, the concentrate form) contains an abundance of these cystine residues, thus making it a powerful immunomodulator against cancer, toxins, infections, or any other bodily insult.

Animals that were fed whey protein concentrate showed dramatic enhancement in immune response to various pathogens and extreme cancer-causing chemicals. Whey protein concentrate fights cancer. In testing whey, animals were fed whey protein concentrate and were then exposed to a powerful carcinogen known as dimethythydrazine. They were able to sustain a far more vigorous immune response to this cancer-causing chemical than animals fed any other type of protein. Also, tumors were smaller and the numbers of tumors were far fewer in the whey protein fed animals.

Supporting this notion of whey being protective against cancer was a startling study published by the American Association for Cancer Research. In this study whey protein was compared to soy protein and casein (a low order of milk protein). The article concluded, "whey appears to be at least twice as effective as soy in reducing both tumor incidence and multiplicity." This is news of staggering proportions and profound ramifications when choosing between soy protein and whey protein.

Furthermore, the same "cysteine donor" effect unique to whey protein and not found in soy that seems to be at work in preventing cancer has recently been demonstrated to enhance muscular performance and decrease muscular fatigue. Another study concluded that "prolonged supplementation with a product designed to augment antioxidant defenses resulted in improved volitional performance."

If all that wasn't enough, consider that whey protein increases the life span of animals. Several studies using whey protein concentrate have shown increases in life span. Mice that were fed whey protein concentrate lived an average of 30-percent longer than mice fed standard lab chow or casein.

Because of increased bioavailability (over whole intact protein), solubility properties, and concentration of branch chain amino acids (23%), whey protein isolates are the superior form of protein supplementation. As additional benefits of whey protein are documented, the popularity of this amazing supplement will continue to grow. For the knowledgeable consumer and health enthusiast, there should be no mystery or controversy when it comes to choosing whey as the primary protein source. These research findings, combined with continuous study on whey protein, should convince anyone that whey protein is truly *the* life-extension, health-promoting protein.

In summary, the popularity of whey protein continues to grow, and rightfully so. While a considerable body of research supports its use, compelling evidence continues to mount reinforcing whey as the best all-purpose protein source of preference for the human body, and thus, the protein of choice for those on the Greenwich Diet.

Seven Basic Protein Rules of the Greenwich Diet

1. Predominantly whey protein, but also whole eggs or egg whites, skim milk, lean steak, chicken breast and fish.
2. Absolutely no ham, bacon, or other pork products (nitrates and nitrites).
3. Absolutely no soy or soy products unless carefully screened and taken in small amounts as a medicinal food and not as a source of protein.
4. 50 percent of all protein should consist of whey protein (preferably a powder of 85 percent or greater concentration). This makes meals small and extremely convenient.
5. Minimum protein intake of 0.8 grams per pound of body weight for non-exercisers, up to 1.3 grams per pound of body weight for heavy exercisers.
6. Protein meals should consist of between 20 and 30 grams per feeding.
7. Protein meals should be spaced throughout the day by 2.5 to 3.0 hours for non-exercisers and 2.0 to 2.5 hours for exercisers.

Fat

The Skinny on Fat

The excessive saturated fat content in our diet has been linked closely to some of the most serious diseases, specifically heart disease, stroke and cancer. It is rare these days not to have heard of the recommendations to decrease your intake of saturated fat. Many of us are making efforts to cut down on consumption of pork, cold cuts, sausage, bacon, hot dogs, cheeses, butter, ice cream, sour cream and whole milk products. Unfortunately, a total ban on fat in the diet is a big mistake because there are some fats that are needed in your diet and, in fact, very healthy.

Unlike animal fats, polyunsaturated fats are derived from vegetables and remain liquid at room temperature. For several decades, polyunsaturated fats have been considered the more healthy fats. We have been urged by the food industry, the media and even our doctors to use margarine and vegetable shortening (corn, safflower, soy and sunflower oils) instead of butter and lard. We are reminded that polyunsaturated fats are cholesterol-free and very low in saturated fat. However, it is ironic that in recent years we've learned that even these vegetable fats and oils are linked to obesity, cancer and heart disease and that we therefore need to discriminate even further.

It is unfortunate that much of the nutritional information available today fails to mention the essential fatty acids. Again, as with amino acids, the word "essential" refers to the inability of the body to manufacture the nutrient and the necessity to obtain it through the diet. The two essential fatty acids, and the ones focused on by Greenwich Dieters, are polyunsaturated fatty acids (PUFAs). One is alpha-linolenic acid (an omega-3 fatty acid, or "n-3"), and the other is linoleic acid (an omega-6 fatty acid, or "n-6"). These two types of PUFAs must be considered separately because they are metabolically and functionally distinct.

Beginning with the alpha-linolenic acid (n-3), the first and most important consideration is recognizing that n-3 obtained through the diet is not particularly metabolically active until it undergoes a labor intensive and often energetically unfavorable conversion to two metabolically active forms. These forms are eicosapentaenoic acid (EPA) and docosahexaenoic acid (DHA), which are found in great amounts in fish and fish oils (i.e., mostly cold-water fish), but also in rabbits and wild game in small amounts. Taking in only alpha-linolenic acid requires a conversion to EPA and DHA through a fairly complex, multi-step biochemical reaction. This inefficient conversion makes a diet that is sufficiently high in alpha-linolenic acid but low in supplemental EPA and DHA actually insufficient to meet one's health needs. Although plant sources of alpha-linolenic acid are useful (i.e., flaxseed oil contains more than 50 percent alpha-linolenic acid by weight), the preference in supplementation for Greenwich Dieters are EPA and DHA from fish oils.

Like alpha-linolenic acid, linoleic acid (n-6) is important and essential, as well. However, most people actually seem to get far too much n-6 in their diets. You see, as I mentioned, humans have evolved from a primordial level with much healthier nutrients. They relied heavily on a diet with a balance of n-3 to n-6 fatty acids. As such, this balance has been incorporated into our genetics. We now have a pre-programmed need to have an equal, one-to-one ratio of n-3 to n-6 fatty acids in our diet. With time, though, modern diets have come to rely on processed food, excessive carbohydrates, cooking oils and lard, to name a few. The result has been a grossly disproportionate imbalance of n-3 to n-6. Some data quote the ratio as being as lopsided as one-to-25 in some areas.

So, if you're thinking cap is on, you might be wondering why, if both n-3 and n-6 are essential and must be obtained through the diet, there's no problem with too much n-6 as long as your getting a high enough level of n-3. Well, the answer is quite simple. An n-3 deficiency is accentuated when n-6 is elevated beyond that one-to-one ratio because this excessive concentration inhibits the synthesis of DHA from alpha-linolenic acid. Thus, diets rich in corn, safflower and sunflower oils (all low in n-3 and high in n-6) can lead to n-3 deficiency. Remember, the converse is not true. You don't have to worry about an excess of n-3, especially in the form of EPA and DHA. Herein is the reason the Greenwich Diet is so heavy on supplemental fish oils.

With all that explained, just what in general are the benefits of these healthy fats? They are cardioprotective and ease the passage of blood and blood constituents through the coronary arteries. They have anti-arrhythmic effects and can protect the heart from potentially fatal rhythms. They can reduce blood clotting and thrombosis nearly everywhere in the body. They are converted to hormones (i.e., prostaglandin E-3, for example) that can lower blood pressure, serve as a diuretic and rid the body of excess water, exert a positive effect on the immune and nervous systems, and enhance efficient digestion and absorption by stimulating gastric secretions and natural smooth-muscle contraction. As such, I have found in my practice that fish oil supplementation has been successful in treating innumerable cases of constipation, as well as aiding in the alleviation of elevated triglycerides, skin disorders, arthritis, allergies and unexplained hair loss (alopecia).

Five Basic Fat Rules of the Greenwich Diet:

1. Limit an excess of "direct" animal fat (butter, cream, lard, cheese, fatty meat).
2. "Indirect" animal fat sources are permissible (fish, lean steak, chicken, eggs, skim milk, game, etc.).
3. Of the vegetable oils, avoid corn, safflower and peanut oil.
4. 1,000 to 3,000 milligrams per day of EPA/DHA gel-cap supplementation for non-exercisers; 2,000 to 5,000 milligrams per day of EPA/DHA gel-cap supplementation for exercisers.
5. Olive oil is the only table oil permitted for cooking and on salads.

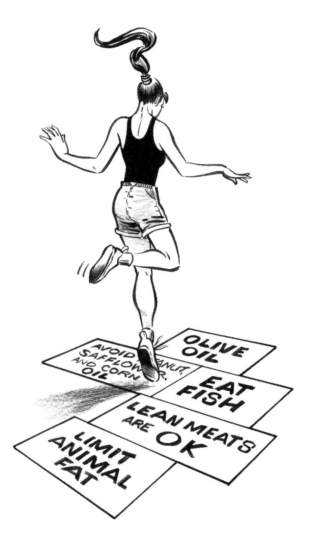

Fiber

Fiber is a unable to be completely digested and absorbed into the bloodstream. In its pure form, it is not used as an energy source by the body and therefore is non-caloric. Fiber is also not a total nutrient because it is unable to nourish the body. However, it is crucial to good health.

Fiber is found in plants. It is the building material that gives plants their strong stems and leaves. These fibers are composed of many sugar units, also known as polysaccharides. However, these sugar units are unable to be digested by the body into simple sugars, which convert into energy, or calories.

There are two types of fibers: soluble and insoluble. Soluble fibers are able to dissolve in water and become gummy or viscous. Soluble fibers help lower blood cholesterol levels and help regulate the body's use of sugars. Soluble fibers are broken down into two classes; one is pectins and the other is gums and mucilages. Pectins are found in apples, carrots, beets, bananas, cabbage, dried peas and okra. Pectin helps slow the absorption of food, allowing sugar to be absorbed more slowly by the bloodstream. This aids in controlling blood sugar levels. Pectin also removes metals and toxins, lowers cholesterol and reduces the risk of heart disease and gallstones. Gums and mucilages are found in oatmeal, oat bran, sesame seeds and dried beans. These soluble fibers also help regulate blood glucose levels, aid in lowering cholesterol, and help in the removal of toxins.

Interestingly, the soluble type of fiber is of much greater importance in diets higher in carbohydrates because of the ability of this type of fiber to positively influence blood sugar. However, with the Greenwich Diet so relatively low in carbohydrates, elevated blood sugar and diabetes are far less of a concern. Thus, the emphasis on fiber favors the insoluble type.

Insoluble fiber, also known as "roughage," is a powerful anticarcinogen and digestive aid. This type of fiber gives structure to plant cell walls and includes cellulose, hemicellulose and lignin. Cellulose is a nondigestible carbohydrate found in the outer layer of fruits and vegetables, including carrots, broccoli, peas, green beans, beets, Brazil nuts and lima beans. Cellulose helps aid in the removal of cancer-causing substances from the colon wall, and helps prevent constipation, colitis, hemorrhoids and varicose veins. Hemicellulose is a nondigestible fiber that absorbs water, cabbage, peppers, various green vegetables and beets. Hemicellulose aids in weight loss, helps prevent constipation, may prevent colon cancer and helps control carcinogens in the intestinal tract. Lignin is a form of fiber that helps lower cholesterol, prevents gallstone formation by binding with bile acids, and is beneficial for those with diabetes or colon cancer. It is found in significant amounts in carrots, green beans, peas, Brazil nuts and tomatoes.

Fiber-rich foods are usually bundled with nutrients, vitamins, minerals and phytochemicals, all of which help in preventing cancer, heart disease and diabetes. Most foods with significant amounts of fiber, such as leafy greens and broccoli, are packed with essential nutrients. For example, many vegetables contain antioxidant vitamins, such as beta-carotene and vitamin C, which may help protect against cancer. Eating plenty of fiber over many years helps prevent colon and rectal cancers. The cause of colon cancer is uncertain. However, about 25 years ago, scientists noted that these cancers were more common in Western countries where people ate less fiber.

The high-fiber Greenwich Diet may help reduce the risk of cancer in two ways: 1. By speeding the time it takes for waste to pass through the digestive tract, and 2. By forming a bulkier, heavier stool. If food waste moves slowly through the digestive tract, there is more time for potentially harmful substances to come in contact with the intestinal wall. Bulkier stools can actually help dilute the concentration of these harmful substances.

Fiber-rich foods make up a large part of the Greenwich Diet because these foods are healthy, low in saturated fat, fairly filling, and so often low in total calories. Because they take longer to chew, you tend to eat less, and with their added bulk they help fill you up. Also, fiber contains a negligible amount of calories and people tend to lose body fat.

A typical American diet supplies only about half the amount of fiber the body needs, averaging about 11 grams daily. That really is not much and should be increased considering all the beneficial outcomes fiber can have on the body. Women typically eat more fiber than men do, but have other problems when it comes to taking in enough protein and water. Overall, however, most adults do not consume as much fiber as they need for their health.

To increase the benefit of fiber, many experts recommend consuming 20-35 grams of fiber daily. Unlike the Recommended Dietary Allowance (RDA) given for various vitamins and minerals, there isn't an RDA for total fiber intake, or for the amounts of soluble and insoluble fiber. The Greenwich Diet supplies approximately 20-50 grams of fiber daily, derived from high fiber, vegetables and salads.

However, don't overdo it. Stick to the guidelines of the Greenwich Diet, because even though fiber is good, there is the possibility of consuming too much. Eating more than 50 grams of fiber daily can lead to problems. Such an extreme regimen may decrease the amount of vitamins and minerals your body absorbs, among them zinc, iron, magnesium and calcium. Too much fiber can also move food too quickly through the intestines causing an interference in the absorption of vital nutrients.

When increasing your fiber intake, make sure to also increase your water or other fluid intake. Fiber acts like a sponge in the colon preventing constipation and other related intestinal problems. Fiber holds onto water and keeps waste moving through the intestine. Therefore, adequate fluid intake is necessary for fiber to do its job properly. Aim for satisfying the Greenwich Diet guidelines for water intake as well as fiber.

Be careful about relying on supplemental fiber and not on natural fiber from food. Depending on the type of supplement, fiber pills or powders won't make a significant difference to your health, although it may help relieve constipation. Most fiber supplements contain minimal amounts of fiber when compared to the amount found in high-fiber foods. Those fiber supplements with more fiber may inhibit the absorption of some minerals, which can cause problems for people whose diets are nutrient-deficient. People who do take fiber supplements daily may eventually become reliant on them. So, suffice to say that natural fiber, and not fiber supplements, are acceptable to the Greenwich Diet.

A Fiber Philosophy

I believe the elimination of fiber in the American diet is a major factor responsible for premature aging and chronic diseases. A diet rich in fiber will promote optimal transit time in the gastrointestinal tract. Healthy Greenwich Diet fiber is what we call "insoluble" fiber. As such, it occupies space in the gastrointestinal tract and pushes all contents through with speed. It is for this reason that fiber helps prevent constipation, straining, hemorrhoids, fissures, appendicitis and an overgrowth of undesirable intestinal bacteria. And with all the concern about cancer causing carcinogens, it also helps to avoid letting anything you've eaten sit around and fester in your intestines just waiting to grow some fungating mass. Fiber keeps such toxins from getting a foothold simply by speeding digested foods along, eliminating "loitering" in your colon.

Healthy, regular bowel movements are not only rewarding for many (i.e., just look at your cat race across the room after he uses the pan!) but also create normal pressure within the intestines and the abdominal cavity. This prevents diseases like diverticulosis, diverticulitis, and hiatal hernia.

A fiber-rich diet will make for a healthy environment in the body so that the more favorable bacteria (lactobacilli) are formed and unfavorable toxin-producing bacteria and yeast won't flourish.

Fiber stimulates the secretion of pancreatic enzymes and bicarbonate. Such substances prevent incompletely digested proteins from reaching the colon. A fiber-rich diet also prevents gallstones by increasing bile solubility. The binding and diluting of other carcinogenic bile acids also prevents colorectal cancer. Perhaps one of the most important benefits of fiber for many is its ability to bind and excrete cholesterol. In addition, fiber can even bind heavy metals and toxins, thus protecting the body from harm.

Examples of Greenwich Diet fibers include lettuce, spinach, celery, carrots, broccoli, asparagus, cauliflower, Brussels sprouts and spinach. Examples of fibers that are carbohydrate-based foods and thus not on the Greenwich Diet include bread, pasta, rice, potatoes, corn, rye, beans, lentils, barley, legumes and fruits.

Water

Water is the most common substance on the planet and, I believe, the most neglected of all essential nutrients. It also happens to be the most abundant substance in the human body (a well-known fact that far too many health-care professionals ignore). On average, an adult's body weight is nearly 70 percent water. This corresponds to about twelve gallons. Of course, this specific percentage varies depending on body composition, age and gender, among other factors, but the point remains the same—water is essential. Yet, despite this evidence, I find that far too many people are dehydrated.

Body Composition as a Model for Hydration

Body composition refers to all the substances that make up your body. As pointed out, water occupies by far the greatest portion of what is you. Despite this fact, it is often neglected.

We should look at our body compositions (what we are made up of) as a model for what we consume. Since the body is made up of an enormous amount of water, followed by muscle, fat and trace carbohydrates and elements, our diet should reflect this composition. In so doing, we should correspondingly take in sizable amounts of water along with good portions of protein, fat and fiber, while keeping carbohydrates to a minimum.

Lean muscle contains much more water compared to body fat. Thus, the more muscle you have and the leaner you are, the higher the proportion of water in your body. Males typically have more muscle than females and thus carry a higher percentage of water in their bodies.

Also, this model works in terms of expanding to include mimicking a youthful body. Water accounts for about 75 percent of a newborn's weight, while this amount decreases in the elderly to about 55 percent water weight. As we age, our bodies dry out. Our total body water goes down and our skin becomes dry and cracked. Sadly, although our bodies are in desperate need of hydration as we age, we tend to drink less, thus compounding our problems. So, you lose water as you get older. Get it? Don't get old before your time. Drink.

Dehydration = Disease

Water contains no calories, yet every cell, tissue and organ, and almost every life-sustaining body process, needs water to function. Water transports nutrients and oxygen to your body cells and carries waste products out of the cells. It lubricates body tissues. Water moistens your mouth, eyes and nose. Water makes up the tissues that cushion your joints and protect your body organs. Water is also the main constituent of all body fluids, including blood, gastric (stomach) juice, saliva, amniotic fluid (for a developing fetus) and urine.

The value of proper hydration cannot be underestimated. In fact, whenever someone becomes sick and is brought to the hospital, be it for fever, infection, trauma, blood loss, or whatever, the first thing that is almost always done on nearly every patient is to set up an intravenous. The majority of time we end up giving the person fluids. When faced with severe illness, the hydration of the patient is a first consideration for the physician when a life is at stake. Thus, it should come as no surprise that this should be a first consideration for you as well. Dehydration can result from a disease process or result in a disease process.

Obesity is considered to be a disease. But, quite frankly, in my experience, being even moderately overweight can lead to problems and ailments. Interestingly, while I believe the majority of Americans are not adequately hydrated, many of these same people are overweight. Is there a connection? I believe there is. In fact, I believe that this may be the primary reason so many people fail to lose weight on any diet. Whatever the type of caloric restriction or physical activity, the body only gives up fat in a healthy way when all nutrient requirements including water are satisfied. Thus, if the body is, in essence, traumatized by not having enough fluid, you can't expect it to allow you to lose fat. Your body simply won't let you do it easily.

Water During Exercise

To keep your body functioning normally and to avoid dehydration, your body needs a continuous water supply. During exercise it is common to lose water, especially on a hot, humid day. Losing one or two pounds of your body's water weight can create a feeling of thirst. With more fluid loss, strength will fade. With even more water loss, you will suffer heat exhaustion or possibly heat stroke.

The amount of water your body needs each day usually

depends on the amount of energy your body uses. Climate and level of activity also affect the need for water. For example, your body uses more water to maintain its normal temperature when exposed to extreme temperatures, whether hot or cold. With strenuous work or exercise, your body loses water through perspiration.

The Choice is Water

Drinking pure water should satisfy fluid requirements. Some other beverages are okay, but be careful of those sports drinks loaded with high fructose corn syrup. It's a big carbohydrate blast and must be taken into account.

The best choice in terms of what to drink to get in your fluids is just plain water.

Water For Women

Women are particularly negligent in the area of keeping themselves well hydrated. In my practice, I have noticed through physical examination and careful history, although quite common among men, there is a far greater number of women who are nothing short of parched. It wasn't until fairly recently that I learned the most likely reason for this skew. A female patient came in for a routine doctor visit. It became obvious that she took little time to hydrate herself adequately throughout the day. She wasn't the first, nor will she be the last, dehydrated and extreme-ly busy middle-aged professional woman in a high stress job that seeks consultation. The difference with this visit was the contribution of her own insight.

She explained, "women have it tougher than men when it comes to using the bathroom. While men can relieve themselves almost anywhere, women often have to sit. It matters what you sit on, don't you think?" I agreed, and listened carefully as she went on. "As a woman, going to the bathroom is a big deal. As a man, you don't realize it. Men are in and out of the bathroom. In public, at restaurants, parties, clubs and even department stores women have to wait in line. It's no wonder I avoid the water fountain most of the time." I thanked her for her honesty; I simply hadn't perceived this problem.

Couple this with a high-stress, busy day in which you are being pulled in a million different directions, and it is easy to see how hydration is overlooked. However, this doesn't change the fact that your body must receive adequate hydration or your health will suffer. As amazing as the body is, you simply cannot "compensate" for not having enough fluid by "getting used to" avoiding water.

THE GREENWICH DIET vs. FIVE OTHER POPULAR DIETS
A Head-to-Head Comparison

Atkins

My colleague Robert Atkins, M.D., took an awful lot of "heat" from the medical community when he first introduced this diet. In fact, the diet is still viewed by many conservative physicians as "dangerous." Nonetheless, although quite different in many ways from the Greenwich Diet, I find Dr. Atkins' approach fascinating and profound in many ways.

Considered by many to be the ultimate ketogenic diet, Atkins advocates a radical restriction of carbohydrate consumption with a host of specific nutritional supplements. Individuals on the Atkins diet are told to monitor their carbohydrate intake for two weeks while consuming high amounts of protein and low carbohydrates to determine the level of carbohydrate intake conducive to weight loss. In this diet, carbohydrate intake may be as high as 60 grams per day, or as low as 15 grams, depending on the individual.

Although the Greenwich Diet is quite similar to the

Atkins Diet in terms of carbohydrate intake, the biggest differences are in protein and fat. The Atkins diet advocates soy protein. This is in sharp contrast to the Greenwich Diet, which is whey protein-based. Again, it is my belief that soy is a medicinal food for selected individuals but does not count as dietary protein. Whey, on the other hand, is an incomparable source of protein and far superior to soy.

Also, one of the major criticisms of the Atkins Diet is the constipation it causes. Such a physiologic response is unhealthy. Regular bowel movements are important not only to one's health, but to one's personal comfort as well. This problem does not occur with the Greenwich Diet because of the heavy emphasis on high fiber and good hydration (regular water drinking). Unlike so many Atkins dieters, Greenwich Dieters are simply not constipated. Atkins has classically considered many vegetables to be carbohydrates and thus avoided in your diet. The Greenwich Diet classifies most vegetables not as carbohydrates, but as fiber-based healthy foods loaded with phytonutrients. Thus, not only are they acceptable, but they actually form a major part of the Greenwich Diet foods.

In terms of the biggest criticism, fat, again the difference between the Atkins and Greenwich diets is self-evident. Atkins basically believes you can eat as much fat as you want while eliminating carbohydrates. This includes animal fat and lard. This has raised a great deal of concern about the Atkins Diet being unhealthy over the long-term. Butter, bacon, greasy sausages and pork rinds are all okay! Sorry, but that doesn't fly in the Greenwich Diet. As such,

I consider the Greenwich Diet to be a healthier version of the Atkins approach. Although the Greenwich Diet allows for a relatively high amount of fat, the source is predominantly from fish oil, with some olive oil as well. Unlike pig fat and lard, which can lead to clogging of the vessels in the heart, the fats found in the Greenwich Diet are actually heart-healthy and promote favorable lipid levels in the blood. But really, do I have to work very hard to convince you that Atkins is wrong in thinking that eating greasy pig is good for you?

40-30-30/Zone

Developed by non-physicians, this dietary prescription involves eating meals in order to maximize the burning of body fat for energy through hormonal control (i.e., minimizing insulin surges by limiting sugar in the diet, while maximizing glucagon). It is a very clever idea and, like Atkins who came before them, credit should be given to these visionaries who boldly went against the grain by targeting carbohydrates as a major problem.

Each meal contains 40 percent of the calories from predominantly low-glycemic carbohydrates, with 30 percent high-quality protein and 30 percent fat. The avoidance of carbohydrates in the Greenwich Diet reflects the emphasis, although more stringently than in the 40-30-30 diet. However, the divergence of beliefs takes place with the notion by the 40-30-30 proponents that there are really no good or bad foods. Rather, the key is to achieve proper balance of the foods you eat. An attractive idea, but unfortunately, with what we know about cancer-causing carcinogenic foods, preservatives, nitrates, nitrites, dyes, chemicals and saturated fats, to name a few, "balance" notions are a bit too simplistic.

In terms of fat, many 40-30-30 proponents tend to believe that as long as no more or less than 30 percent of your diet comes from fat, you are fine, regardless of the fat source. In sharp contrast, the Greenwich Diet puts great value on obtaining the right kind of fat in the diet. In fact, Greenwich Dieters rely heavily on minimizing saturated animal fat and lard, while maximizing the healthy fats from fish oil and olive oil. Some 40-30-30 literature refers to obtaining three varieties of fat in equal proportions (10 percent saturated, 10 percent unsaturated, and 10 percent mono-unsaturated). Again, the proportion and balance idea is an appealing one, but, unlike the rather brilliant logic behind the 40-30-30 minimization of carbohydrates for purposes of keeping insulin in check, there appears to be very little other reasoning for this approach.

Perhaps the biggest difference between the Greenwich Diet and 40-30-30 is that the 40-30-30 diet still clearly requires you to take in nearly as much carbohydrate as protein. Again, in sharp contrast, the Greenwich Diet offers quite a bit more latitude in eating far more proteins than carbohydrates, and in particular, whey protein. With all we know about the superiority of whey protein, the Zone diet never even mentions it.

Ornish

Dr. Dean Ornish has developed two diets: the Reversal Diet and the Prevention Diet. The advantage of these diets is that they are heart healthy and do seem to actually reverse coronary disease. However, for overall health, it is my steadfast belief that his approach is greatly flawed.

The Reversal Diet is a vegetarian diet. In particular, the heavy emphasis on carbohydrates (i.e., 70 to 75 percent carbohydrates), with no restriction on total caloric intake, makes this what I call a "narcotic diet." Loading up on carbohydrates dramatically limits the amount of protein and healthy fat you can take in. Remember, only certain types of protein and fat are scientifically proven to be essential. Carbohydrates are not. Doesn't that tell you something? Clearly, protein and fat are essential because of their role in health and well-being. Any good diet is going to focus on maximizing what is essential and minimizing what is filler. Carbohydrates, on the other hand, are the narcotic. As such, the Ornish approach only allows for 10 percent fat (most polyunsaturated or monounsaturated) and a paltry 15 to 20 percent protein.

Of course, with a high fiber approach and a limit of five milligrams of cholesterol daily, it is hardly a surprise that the diet is heart-healthy. But, I believe it is little else. Emphasizing a limit on alcohol consumption (under two ounces per day), excluding MSG, and allowing only moderate use of table sugar are probably good things.

The Prevention Diet follows the same basic guidelines

with slight alterations. If basic conditions are not met (cholesterol of under 150, good ratio of total cholesterol to HDL) the diet should begin by eating 20 percent fat (doubling amount of fat recommended in the Reversal Diet). After eight weeks, if there is no reduction in cholesterol to the target level of 150, more foods high in saturated fats and cholesterol can be eliminated. If, after another eight weeks, the target level has not been achieved through diet alone, exercise and stress reduction is implemented. Finally, cholesterol-lowering medications will be introduced if the levels are not reduced.

Again, although a step up in terms of overall health, the prevention version is little better than the reversal version in terms of systemic benefit. I find these approaches extremely narrow and it wouldn't surprise me if, while you're apparently reversing your coronary disease with high fiber and low saturated fat, you are exposing your body to illness down the road by neglecting essential amino acids and fatty acids. I believe the Greenwich Diet, which gives you a ton of fiber, protein and healthy fat (fish and olive oil), can provide the same benefits of the Ornish approach without sacrificing essential nutrients. Contrary to the proponents, I don't think the Ornish approach is the best road to health and wellness. Of course, almost anything is better than the standard American diet!

Pritikin

The crux of the Pritikin Diet is based on the principle of extremely low fat content. This diet restricts not only saturated fats; it bans all fats, including the unsaturated fats from vegetables, nuts and seeds. No need to belabor the point, but with all we now know about the benefits of healthy fats, this approach is nothing short of ignorant. Although archaic in the extreme, this diet still warrants mentioning because of its continued popularity.

The rules here are pretty simple. Only 10 percent of the day's total calories should come from fat (no more than 34 percent from poultry and fish and 15 percent or less for all other foods). Pritikin proponents modify the daily number of complex carbohydrates plus the total numbers of fruit servings to equal the total number of vegetable servings each day. They say you should avoid eating any carbohydrates and fruits until you've eaten all eight vegetable servings for the day. (Is your brain hurting trying to figure this out?) In addition, they like so-called "preferred carbohydrates" (the obvious antithesis of the Greenwich Diet—we never "prefer" carbohydrates). The clear preference toward making carbohydrates the focus of the Pritikin Diet violates the central teaching of the Greenwich Diet and I believe it is deeply flawed.

It seems the only good things about the diet include a reduction in consumption of refined foods (two out of eight servings can be refined), an emphasis on more frequent feedings (five to six small meals and snacks daily), and a limitation on calories after dinner. Other than those principles, it is difficult to extract any sane take-home lessons from this diet.

Scarsdale

The Scarsdale Diet, consistent with the Greenwich Diet, involves high protein and relatively low carbohydrates. The diet also advocates drinking fluids (at least four glasses of water or diet soda per day), although less than the Greenwich Diet. Proponents advocate spicing food with additions such as herbs, salt, pepper, lemon, vinegar, Worcestershire sauce, soy sauce mustard and ketchup.

Unfortunately, divergence from the Greenwich Diet comes in the form of far too little healthy fat, including maintaining a tolerance for pork. Another feeble concept this diet clings to is the "three square meal" idea. Eating smaller meals with much higher frequency throughout the day is the hallmark of the Greenwich Diet and one of the keys to health and sustained loss of body fat.

DIETARY SUPPLEMENTS

VI

Why Use Dietary Supplements?

What can we do to change the sickly and often deadly pattern we've fallen into as a society? One answer lies within the framework of the Greenwich Diet. Dietary supplementation along with the proper vital natural nutrient foods is the path to wellness.

If we are to advance as a society, we cannot be ignorant. We must embrace a smarter way of living. Supplementing our diets makes sense because supplementation helps us avoid disease and illness prior to seeing these conditions manifest in our bodies. Supplements are good preventive care.

Intelligent physicians no longer scoff at the idea of taking vitamins. The truth is, many of my colleagues, including the skeptics, actually take some form of vitamin but are actually reluctant to recommend these same supplements to their patients! It baffles me. Well, the tide is turning. Evidence that vitamin and mineral supplementation can reduce the risk of disease, and actually cure disease, is rapidly mounting. Vitamin E has been clearly indicated as an aid to prevent prostate and colon cancer, as well as reduce the risk of cardiovascular disease. Studies confirm the importance of calcium and vitamin D in reducing the risk of osteoporosis. Supplemental folic acid for women reduces the occurrence and recurrence of newborn neural tube defects, as well as decreasing the risk of heart disease in older adults. Vitamin C has been shown to reduce the risk of bladder cancer. Selenium has shown great promise as a preventive aid in a host of various cancers.

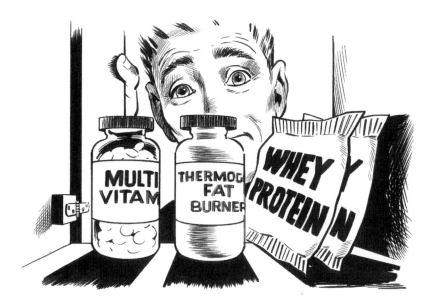

The bottom line is that we have control over the future of our health simply by making the right choices when it comes to our bodies' nourishment. The problem is that, returning to the primordial example of early man, we no longer spend our days foraging for food. Instead, we sit at our desks pushing papers or glued to the Internet. Many ages ago food was the only major need, so nourishing oneself throughout the day was a given. Today, our complicated lives have introduced so many concerns that we have moved far away from the simple life of nourishing our bodies throughout the day. Business success and money woes have taken the place of making feeding a priority. But our hard-driving ambitions for personal success and our preoccupation with our own minds and the minds of others, simply doesn't change the fact that our bodies need to be properly fed. Over the past million or so years—and regardless of what skeletons tell us—there has been a greater evolution of the mind than of the body.

Since the Greenwich Diet requires frequent feedings, in our lives full of many concerns and distractions, it is virtually impossible to expect healthy dietary compliance without some easier way. Thus, the recommendation by the American Dietetic Association to obtain nutrients from a wide variety of foods in order to maintain health and reduce the risk of disease is simply unrealistic. The only way we can realistically satisfy this need in both a cost-effective and time-efficient way is to supplement our diets. In addition to eating only when time allows, new supplement technology now permits us to quickly nourish ourselves while on the go and insure that we receive a generous portion of the essentials.

Ignorance Ain't Bliss

Despite all the scientific proof of the effectiveness of dietary supplementation, people are still too slow to become educated and involved in their use. I am always sadly amused to see people who don't believe supplements work, suddenly start exploring the possibilities with an open mind as soon as they fall ill. It's at that point I find that close-minded people suddenly have a refreshingly attentive disposition. Unfortunately, for more serious illnesses, it is often too late for even the best supplement regimens to effectively counter what is ailing them.

But this skepticism is hardly restricted to the average consumer. It has always been a struggle to convince my fellow physicians of the extreme value and importance of dietary supplementation. In fact, I find that the majority of my physician colleagues won't acknowledge the value of dietary supplementation in the daily maintenance and promotion of a healthy and disease-free body. It is this narrow thinking from health care professionals that contributes so negatively to the way we, as a society, view the inevitability of being overweight, aging and suffering from illness.

As physicians, our biggest "malfunction" is that we feed into what I call a disease-based model of thinking. As is reflected in the way we are trained, we typically wait for people to be sick, debilitated and even hospitalized before we address their needs. We are not trained as much on how to keep people healthy, well, and disease-free. Physicians, along with far too many other health care professionals, tend to be most comfortable addressing diseases and illness. Since this wellness-based model I preach is not the standard, I find few of my colleagues adept at keeping their patients lean, energetic, healthy, and disease-free. In fact, while my patients thrive, others survive.

Your average physician visit can last as little as a few minutes. How can you be a good listener in a few minutes? A good listener means allowing someone to speak more than two sentences. Most patients are very interested in dietary supplements but are hesitant to ask their doctors. Although they won't admit it, many physicians believe that if you are not sick, your body doesn't need much attention. It's a crazy way thinking.

It is for this reason that, according to most people, the doctor is the person you go to only when you're sick. Perpetuating this model, many physicians believe they must have all of the answers for their patients who are ill, but they are too hesitant to explore new ideas on prevention. Unreasonable physicians hate admitting when they don't know something. On the other hand, progressive physicians are quick to admit when they don't have an answer and are open to new ideas.

The truth behind this reluctance is that many doctors, apart from unfounded and conditioned skepticism when it comes to dietary supplements, simply lack a knowledge of dietary nutrients. Thus, too many fail to recognize the incredible power all of us have to take control of our health by simply making the proper supplement choices and taking needed nutrients into our bodies.

We physicians are a curious bunch. We rely heavily on medical and scientific journals regarding so many disease-oriented subjects. But when it comes to vitamins, minerals and other supplements, it's as if we ignore the published information. For example, vitamin E and the prevention of cardiovascular disease, colon cancer and prostate cancer; folic acid for a healthy heart; calcium and vitamin D for osteoporosis; and, more recently, lycopenes from tomatoes as a cancer-preventing agent. These are just a few associations that only scratch the surface of what we know and what has been demonstrated scientifically. Any way you look at it, one thing is certain. Supplementing the diet is a healthy thing to do.

When I look back on my personal experience as a state assistant medical examiner, I can't begin to tell you how many deaths I've been called to investigate, that, despite what I listed as the official, accepted cause of death—a heart attack, stroke, cancer, or whatever—I believe originated from years of making bad dietary choices and neglecting key nutrients.

Being overweight means whether you are conscious of it or not, vital nutrients are being ignored. It isn't as simple as, "Hey, you're just eating too much!" In fact, those folks who are overweight are curiously lacking in key nutrients. You'd think these people would have an excess of such nutrients. Wrong. Such individuals typically lack nutrients despite the excessive quantities of food they consume. This is primarily less a result of the amount of food eaten and more a result of the type of food in their diets. The average person's food choices are almost invariably nutrient-poor at some level. Add to that, when attempting to restrict calorie intake in order to lose weight, the average diet encourages the elimination of all the wrong nutrients. It's no wonder ignorance among patients and doctors is widespread. Everyone seems confused. People on the Greenwich Diet are not.

Aging, Illness, and Immunity

There are numerous theories about why we age and become ill. But perhaps the one that has received the most attention explains this degenerative process in terms of oxidation and free radical production causing DNA damage and cellular destruction. In primeval times, most living organisms were "anaerobic." That is, their respiratory systems did not have oxygen available and therefore did not require it. Energy production in this way was, and is, a relatively simple pathway. It is deemed simple because it requires no special cellular organelle to make use of the oxygen molecule. This cellular organelle is called a "mitochondria" and is required to utilize oxygen for energy. If you do not intend to drive very far, you certainly don't need much gas. Think of the mitochondria as the gas station of the cell.

Far less complicated, anaerobic cellular metabolism (those cells not requiring a mitochondria) produce exponentially less energy than aerobic metabolism. Thus, although these cells can survive without oxygen, they can only accomplish very minimal tasks.

But in a world with oxygen readily available, eventually

evolution took hold and the living world witnessed a proliferation of higher life forms that relied predominantly on the much more efficient aerobic respiration.

With all of this in mind, although the utilization of aerobic metabolism for energy is significantly more sensible from the standpoint of evolution to higher life forms, the utilization of oxygen is not without consequence. Oxygen itself degrades into electronically unstable and reactive oxidants that strive to achieve a stable configuration by removing electrons from the molecules of surrounding cell tissue. In so doing, damage results in the liberation of a charged molecule.

This negatively charged particle is liberated in the form of an electron. The release of this free radical by oxygen is a process called oxidation. Anytime a substance loses an electron, oxidation has occurred, and when a cell is stripped of its electrons, the cell itself begins to show instability and impaired function. The result is that cellular aging ensues in a spiral toward cellular death.

Unfortunately, the damage does not end there. As the cell expires, it releases its own set of harmful, charged particles, which in turn exert damage to neighboring cells. This occurs in such a way that a chain reaction of aging and death is triggered at the cellular level.

The evolutionary chain of life has kept this process in check with the emerging of higher organisms equipped with the ability to marginally suppress the damaging effects of reactive oxidants. Humankind stands at the apex of this chain. The human body can effectively harness the immense efficiency of aerobic cellular metabolism while coping with the toxic side effects of oxygen-induced damage. This is accomplished by way of a special system that scavenges harmful free radicals.

Perhaps because cell aging and death is so closely linked to the aerobic liberation of free radicals and the subsequent damage they cause to neighboring cells, it seems to make perfect sense to think that aging and disease in the body are also linked to this process. Herein lies the reason the Greenwich Diet is so incredibly high in antioxidants. From whey protein and its ability to increase cell GSH concentration (a powerful intracellular antioxidant) to the vitamins and other supplements I suggest, you will see a definite preference toward substances that can act as antioxidants.

It is difficult enough to receive the nutrients we need when we are young, but as we age or become ill, our dietary intake falls and we become even more prone to depletion. Sadly, this comes at a time when our bodies are at the point of greatest need for adequate nutrition. Therefore, high-quality nutrient supplementation is required. Thus, nutrient supplementation may be the single most important intervention to counter the aging process.

Like the mechanism of aging, the mechanism of immunity is no different. Studies have shown that the immune system is closely related to poor health and aging. Good diet alone may not be enough. Supplements are your insurance policy. As most people get older, we see changes in their immune systems. Changes in immunity associated with aging include reduced interleukin-2 production, lymphocyte response, and antibody titer after vaccination. Nutrition is a critical determinant of immunocompetence in all age groups. Unfortunately, the average diet barely provides the proper dietary allowance of calcium, magnesium, the B-vitamins and vitamin E, just to name a few. Good dietary habits coupled with wisely chosen supplements are the key to achieving success in health and wellness.

The Power of Antioxidants

The system of scavenging free radicals by antioxidants is the fundamental house cleaning mechanism of our bodies. Research in nearly every area of major interest, from cancer to infectious diseases, seems to focus on this mechanism. Everything from foods to enzymes, vitamins and minerals are all being closely studied for their antioxidant ability. In addition to playing an essential role in nearly every biochemical reaction that occurs in the human body, antioxidants circulate throughout the system, literally picking up liberated harmful free radicals.

Scientists universally acknowledge the fact that free radical production via oxidation is perpetually ongoing in our bodies. As cells perish, new cells are produced. It is accepted that this is an unavoidable consequence of cellular function at the level of any higher organism. But as cells die in their natural cycle, the free radicals released injure surrounding cells. Tissues and organ systems of the body are invariably affected, thus speeding up the aging process and contributing directly to a multitude of illnesses.

Free radicals can be carcinogenic (causing cancer) and mutagenic (causing mutations). It is for this reason that the Greenwich Diet is so low in potentially harmful and cancer-causing carcinogenic substances. This gives the Greenwich Diet an edge over other diets, since it is not only a fat-burning approach, but also one that is healthy and high in antioxidant power.

An ever-increasing number of scientific investigators and health professionals believe free radicals are a common component of most of the chronic degenerative diseases, premature aging and premature death. With an understanding of the dietary contribution to the free radical process and the antioxidant mechanisms that protect us from this process, we are able to develop specific strategies to further defend our health. Such a strategy is the Greenwich Diet.

The Supplement Revolution

In the last two decades, modern medicine has dramatically altered its attitude about the relationship between diet and health. Today, it has become common knowledge that cancer, heart disease, diabetes and high blood pressure are associated with dietary excesses of calories, saturated fat, refined sugar and food additives. We are beginning to understand that many diseases and deaths are not solely the result of natural aging. We are learning that we are prematurely losing our youth and accelerating the aging process by simply making poor dietary choices and neglecting key nutrients at a time when making even the simplest changes can make a world of difference.

Many of us fail to realize the fact that medical treatment is inadequate for many of our most common and worst diseases. Therefore, the best weapon we have is that of prevention. For the most part, our attention is focused on finding and treating disease, not on teaching us how to avoid disease. As a result, there is a mass movement toward self-care and preventive medicine. This includes healthy eating, supplements and exercise.

Crucial to our antioxidant defense system are dietary nutrients such as vitamins E and C and the minerals selenium and zinc. Interestingly, diets in youth tend to be significantly higher in substances like these. Yet, as we get older and our lives become ever more complicated, the concentrations of these crucial compounds drop dramatically in our diets. Hence, the sense of the supplement revolution. Dietary supplementation allows us to fill this void without sacrificing crucial time and adult efficiency required to navigate our complicated lives.

The body's ability to protect itself from free radicals can be enhanced if you make it a habit to avoid dietary sources of free radicals and prepare your meals wisely. Adherence to Greenwich Diet parameters is part of the equation. But, since your control over dietary free radicals may be suboptimal, to maintain your health it is crucial to take supplemental antioxidant nutrients like whey protein, vitamins C, E, and the minerals selenium and zinc.

There are many good reasons to properly supplement your diet with the substances your body needs, but perhaps none greater than to stay healthy and preserve your youth for as long as humanly possible. In a world where we as a society believe that technology has no limits, ironically, when it comes to our bodies, we have accepted a defeatist attitude. Society believes that aging and illness is inevitable and that we should only try and do something about it when it begins to become a problem. The truth is, new discoveries are made every day lending credence to the idea that we are surrounded with everything we need. It is simply a matter of getting enough of these essential elements to satisfy our bodily needs. A proper selection of vitamins, minerals and macronutrients are what we must have to restore and maintain our health.

It is such a simple solution that it defies those who look for a more complicated panacea. Most people accept the defeat that plagues the mind, only to spread this plague of defeat to the body. Poor quality of life, illness and even death follow those who ignore the body's needs. The Greenwich Diet is a solution I teach as a new way of thinking. Don't be one of the walking time bombs. Set yourself apart. Embrace a better life with the Greenwich Diet and provide yourself with the supplements you need to thrive, not just survive. Such a lifestyle is filled with hope and solutions, with proper supplementation as the key to unlocking your body's potential.

What Supplements to Choose: A Method to the Madness

The tangled and confusing web of dietary supplementation can be difficult to negotiate. Providing your body with the right non-pharmaceutical supplements to complement the natural eating of the Greenwich Diet will best ensure the path to lasting health and wellness. This section focuses on substances that should be combined with the Greenwich Diet and those that I believe are helpful in rapidly eliminating excess fat while maintaining a healthy, disease-free body.

Multivitamin

The first consideration when supplementing is incorporating a high-quality multivitamin into the diet. As with the macronutrients in the Greenwich Diet, when you consume the proper amounts of vitamins and minerals you will begin to feel a balance within you. While I recommended striving toward compliance with the Greenwich Diet, our fast-paced lives and the unpredictable situations that confront us on a daily basis might make macronutrient compliance difficult (particularly with the high vegetable and fiber content of the diet). The result can be deficiencies of vitamins and minerals.

Deficiencies cause symptoms of fatigue, sluggishness, cramping, easy distractibility and immune dysfunction. If left uncorrected long enough, deficiencies will lead to illnesses like cardiovascular disease and cancer. Sadly, most people don't recognize that this is easily corrected. The role of multivitamin supplementation is to ensure our bodies receive adequate amounts of an array of important nutrients.

How does multivitamin supplementation contribute to wellness and health maintenance? A high quality multivitamin supplement is one of the best ways to ensure that you are getting a proper amount of vitamins and minerals, especially when it is not clear what it is your body is lacking. Remember, a good multivitamin is your "insurance policy" for total body wellness. A high-quality supplement of this type provides you with what you miss in the diet, especially if you have a fast-paced life, are under a moderate to high stress level, and are missing healthy meals (which seems like just about everyone I know these days).

While I view daily multivitamin supplementation as a disease preventive measure, a steady flow of nutrients in the form of a daily multivitamin can prove very effective in actually lessening the symptoms of an ailment and begin to reverse a disease process that has begun to manifest itself.

As an example, women are among the individuals in greatest need of multivitamin supplementation. Because women go through various life stages, nutritional needs can change. For example, excessive bleeding during menstruation can warrant iron supplementation. Pregnant or breast-feeding women need increased levels of nutrients such as folic acid, iron and calcium. Although I usually caution against supplementation during pregnancy without careful consultation with a gynecologist, lacking adequate intake of these nutrients can cause infant development to be adversely affected. Daily multivitamin supplementation prior to pregnancy is a good strategy to maintain optimum health and an effective preemptive prevention against complications.

Continuing on in life, after menopause, when women lose the protective effects of estrogen, they tend to become more prone to bone loss and osteoporosis. Thus, apart from possible estrogen replacement therapy, a multivitamin rich in calcium and vitamin D is necessary.

Vegetarians can also greatly benefit from multivitamin supplementation. Although usually they have an adequate intake of trace and ultra-trace minerals, if vegetarians do not consume foods in the right combinations, they easily become deficient in other more major nutrients such as calcium, iron, zinc and B-12, to name several. Thus, a multivitamin rich in these substances fits the bill.

Multivitamin supplementation may also be of benefit to persons who are on medication. Medications often block the absorption of vital nutrients and alter the balance of metabolic pathways. Multivitamin supplementation at times when medications are administered can ensure their absorption and utilization by the body.

The exercising population can perhaps most greatly benefit from a good multivitamin. Exercisers have been shown to have an increased need for nutrients such as the B-vitamins, vitamins A, C and E, along with the minerals iron and calcium. Deficiencies in these nutrients place an increased demand on the immune system, may increase muscle soreness, affect energy metabolism, and may lead to certain anemias and bone degeneration. Replenishment of these nutrients will contribute to improved work and athletic performance. In this population, proper supplementation will help improve and maintain optimal immune function, bone development and tissue formation. Consumption of a multivitamin-mineral supplement for one year has been shown to improve the immune response. Hospitalized patients that were given a supplement of vitamins A, C and E for four weeks showed evidence that their immune systems were stronger than those of a placebo group. Also, the multivitamin supplemented subjects experienced fewer days of infection than the individuals in the placebo group.

In terms of a specific product recommendation, **Twinlab Metabolift Multivitamin** is an optimal daily multivitamin/multimineral supplement that will help ensure that your body is receiving the proper nutrients when following low-calorie or high-protein low-carbohydrate diets. It is rich in calcium (which is necessary when taking in large dosage amounts of protein). It will also "kick start" your metabolism into high gear for maximum weight loss. It incorporates specific nutrients to increase thyroid activity naturally without the nervous jitters associated with stimulant products. Low-calorie and high-protein, low-carbohydrate diets lower T$_3$ (triiodothytonine), the most active thyroid hormone, and basal metabolic rate (BMR, or the number of calories your body burns at rest) when dieting. Twinlab Metabolift Multivitamin is available at most vitamin stores. This supplement provides a way of achieving and maintaining the internal physiologic balance that is so easily thrown off when vital substances are lacking in the diet. Having such a potent daily multivitamin/multimineral, high in antioxidant power, is essential to any good dietary program and an important part of the Greenwich Diet. The individual vitamins and minerals that follow detail some of the important nutrients found in the Metabolift multivitamin.

Vitamin C, also known as ascorbic acid, is a major component of the Metabolift multivitamin. Vitamin C has received much attention in the past few years. Research has shown its ability to help the body fight the common cold and other disorders, including cancer. In addition, this vitamin's antioxidant abilities have been highlighted. Vitamin C prevents free radical damage that can cause accelerated aging, certain types of diseases, cancer and cardiovascular disorders.

Your immune system keeps you safe from getting sick and protects your body from breaking down. Vitamin C can help increase your body's resistance to disease by stimulating the production of infection-fighting lymphocytes, a very important part of your immune system. It has the amazing ability to increase the cellular activity responsible for disposing of harmful bacteria, viral cells and cancer cells. Elderly patients given regular doses of this vitamin have shown enhanced immunity. Men who have been tested have shown a 40 percent lower death rate from heart disease and other causes. Vitamin C shortens the duration of a cold and lessens its intensity. It aids in the body's ability to combat stress. Vitamin C is essential for the proper growth and repair of tissue throughout the human body. We can't store vitamin C in our bodies. Thus, it is difficult to obtain the proper levels of this vitamin without supplementation. A good multivitamin always has a high content of vitamin C.

Like vitamin C, vitamin E is also a valuable antioxidant vitamin that can be found in any good multivitamin supplement. Vitamin E is thought to be the single most powerful antioxidant in defending against harmful free radicals (even more potent an antioxidant than vitamin C). The difference between C and E is that E is a fat-soluble vitamin and can be stored in the body, unlike C, which is water-soluble and thus quickly excreted. Vitamin E is found predominantly in plants, usually in the form of seeds and nuts. Thus, like vitamin C, it is difficult to get sufficient amounts in the diet without supplementing. There are a couple of subtypes of vitamin E, but the most important of these are the tocopherols. The alpha-tocopherol subtype is the most widely distributed of these compounds in nature. Note that the action of vitamin E is intimately related to the body's concentration of selenium. Thus, any quality multivitamin with vitamin E will also have within it a significant amount of selenium, since it is such an important cofactor.

Vitamin D is an extremely important vitamin for maintaining bone density because of vitamin D's role in mineral absorption and bone mineralization. A deficiency of vitamin D can cause rickets in children and osteomalacia and osteoporosis, as well as hypocalcaemia (low levels of calcium in the blood), in adults. A multivitamin containing this supplement along with calcium is beneficial in aiding in the prevention of osteoporosis. But this isn't the only role of vitamin D in the body. Vitamin D, when combined with calcium, has anti-cancer properties. It has also been shown that people who have low levels of vitamin D in their blood have a higher incidence of high blood pressure. This suggests a wider therapeutic role for vitamin D. As such, vitamin D has also been shown to be beneficial in the treatment of psoriasis as well as multiple sclerosis and other immune system disorders.

Sun exposure, lifestyle and skin color, degree of air pollution and geographical latitude all affect the vitamin D that can be made by the body. It is also questionable whether any vitamin D is synthesized during the winter months, or if you store enough of it for use during the winter's sub-optimal sun exposure. Thus, if you rarely spend time in the sun, have dark skin, live in the northern latitudes or in a modern city, avoid dairy products or have liver or kidney disease, you may be somewhat deficient in this vitamin.

Vitamin A is another fat-soluble vitamin predominately found in certain fatty foods. Beta-carotene is a "pro-vitamin" and the precursor form of vitamin A. It is changed in the body to vitamin A. Beta-carotene is found mainly in the colorful fruits and vegetables. This vitamin is best known as essential for proper night vision. Vitamin A also maintains the stability of cell membranes; helps the adrenal gland produce cortisol (an anti-inflammatory hormone); aids in ensuring a normal production of thyroid hormone from the thyroid gland; assists in maintaining the covering of nerve cells; aids in immune system reactions; and helps to manufacture red blood cells. People who supplement with vitamin A in moderate levels have fewer colds and better skin.

In a study conducted in China, where the incidence of esophageal and stomach cancer is high, a supplement containing predominantly beta-carotene along with vitamin E and selenium managed to protect against death by up to 13 percent. Thus, it is reasonable to conclude that a proper multivitamin supplement should contain vitamin A. However, be aware that even high fruit diets seldom provide adequate beta-carotene because you would still need to consume as many as nine fruits a day to satisfy the daily requirement.

Vitamin B1, or thiamin, is a water-soluble vitamin involved in energy transformation, metabolism and nerve conduction. Those people with low energy levels that benefit from thiamin supplementation are usually adults with high levels of stress, alcoholics and some elite athletes. There are no known toxicity levels established for thiamin since, like all water-soluble vitamins, any excess is excreted in the urine. Since the stability of thiamin in food is intimately dependent on cooking time, temperature and method of preparation, supplementation with thiamin makes perfect sense.

Vitamin B2, or riboflavin, is similar to thiamin in that it plays a role in producing energy. Deficiency of riboflavin can be seen in diets low in animal protein and leafy vegetables. Adults with hypothyroidism are often found to have a riboflavin deficiency. This is because the enzyme that converts riboflavin to its coenzyme form in the body is regulated by thyroid hormone. It has been theorized that poor energy and weight problems can stem from a deficiency of riboflavin as it relates to thyroid hormone. Riboflavin can be found in small amounts in a variety of different foods. The best sources of riboflavin are milk and dairy products such as cheddar cheese and cottage cheese. Organ meats and other lean meats are also good sources of this vitamin. Unlike thiamin, riboflavin is fairly stable in the presence of heat, water and when exposed to air. Hence, most riboflavin is not lost during cooking or processing. However, when exposed to sunlight riboflavin easily disintegrates. In response to this, milk products come in specially lined containers designed to protect riboflavin along with other light-sensitive vitamins and minerals.

Vitamin B3, or niacin, is a water-soluble vitamin that helps in the body's release of energy from carbohydrates, proteins and fats. Niacin is thus an important provider of energy for all the cells of the body. Niacin is an effective and proven method in conjunction with diet to treat primary elevated cholesterol, reduce LDL (the potentially harmful form of cholesterol), and raise the HDL (the so-called "good" form of cholesterol). Niacin can also help reduce elevated triglycerides. In addition, niacin has been shown to reduce the risk of a subsequent heart attack in an individual with high cholesterol who has already suffered an episode.

Vitamin B6, or pyridoxine, is necessary for the production of nonessential amino acids, which can then be transformed and incorporated into new cells. Pyridoxine converts the amino acid tryptophan into niacin and serotonin, a neurotransmitter in the human brain. Pyridoxine also regulates the syntheses of gamma-aminobutyric acid (GABA), another essential neurotransmitter in the brain. Given its important role in the central nervous system, one can easily see how inadequate pyridoxine intake can result in brain irregularities such as dementia. Pyridoxine also helps in the production of insulin, hemoglobin and antibodies that fight infections.

An important point for Greenwich Dieters is that the daily requirement for pyridoxine increases with increasing protein needs. Since the Greenwich Diet is relatively high in protein, supplemental pyridoxine is essential. Extra protein intake for women during pregnancy and lactation also requires more pyridoxine. In fact, during the first year of an infant's life, the requirement for pyridoxine increases steadily.

Vitamin B12, or cobalamin, functions in the energy metabolism of all body cells and is an essential component of DNA synthesis. It is especially important in the formation of red blood cells. A cobalamin deficiency can result in anemia, nerve damage, sensitive skin and fatigue. Strict vegetarians who restrict animal products from their diets and the elderly are at greatest risk for a cobalamin deficiency. Elderly who have a cobalamin deficiency are usually characterized by yellow skin tone, a swollen tongue and nerve damage. The role of cobalamin is most notable in the bone marrow, gastrointestinal tract and nervous tissue. It also helps metabolize fat and helps the body use amino acid. It is a water-soluble vitamin that is synthesized in the body from bile and other intestinal secretions, thus making the need for dietary consumption relatively small. Also, since the best sources of cobalamin are animal protein foods such as liver, kidney, milk, fish, eggs and cheese, a dietary deficiency of cobalamin among Greenwich Dieters is virtually impossible. Nonetheless, given its important multi-system role, I always like to see it incorporated in some capacity into a multivitamin.

Folic acid is another B vitamin that I like to see included in any quality multivitamin. Folic acid is found in fairly significant amounts in green leafy vegetables like spinach and broccoli, as well as cereals and grains. Folic acid supplementation is well known for its importance in preventing birth defects in the brain and spinal cord. In addition to this, folic acid contributes to a multitude of essential system functions. A deficiency can result in weakness, anemia and even death. Since dietary deficiency is such a common culprit of insufficient folic acid, a multivitamin supplement that includes folic acid is the best way of getting the necessary amount.

Pantothenic acid, also known as pantothenate, is a substance that stimulates growth. The main function of pantothenic acid is to be converted to coenzyme A (CoA) in the body. In its converted form, pantothenic acid is used in a variety of biological processes involving the metabolism of fats, proteins and carbohydrates and the synthesis of hormones, bile and hemoglobin. Pantothenic acid is also very important for the production of neurotransmitters. Deficiency of pantothenic acid produces headaches, fatigue, insomnia, anxiety and depression. On the positive side, if you are an athlete, moderate dose supplementation with pantothenic acid has shown a benefit for enhancing exercise tolerance. Also of interest is that pantothenic acid aids in wound and scar healing. People who suffer from rheumatoid arthritis tend to have lower blood levels of pantothenic acid. In fact, the lower the levels, the more severe the arthritic symptoms. Supplementing with pantothenic acid relieves the stiffness and pain that often leads to decreased disability. A deficiency, or even a marginal intake of pantothenic acid, can adversely affect many processes within the body; hence I look for it to be included in a multivitamin.

Whey Protein Powder

A whey protein powder is the single most important supplement included in the Greenwich Diet. Believe it or not, Little Miss Muffit had the right idea about eating her curds and whey! Although whey protein's health benefits have only recently been discovered, the medicinal use of whey protein has been in existence since the time of Hippocrates. Two ancient proverbs from the Italian city of Florence support the importance of whey protein. They are: "If you want to live a healthy and active life, drink whey," and "If everyone were raised on whey, doctors would be bankrupt." Definitely accurate.

Whey proteins are found in meal replacement powders, enteral solutions and reduced fat products. Whey protein is rich in branch chain amino acids, lactalbumin and traces of fat. It is the ion exchange and micro filtration that removes the microbes and other impurities, allowing for a purer product. Something for those individuals with lactose intolerance to keep in mind is that the filtration processes allow for the removal of lactose in some forms of whey supplements (i.e., whey protein isolate).

Because of increased bioavailability (over whole intact protein), solubility properties, and concentration of branch chain amino acids (23 percent), whey protein isolates are the superior form of protein supplementation. In ranking whey protein for bioavailability (remember, that's how much your body can absorb), the order of preference should be as follows: whey protein isolate, followed by whey protein concentrate, and then whey protein peptides.

In terms of comparing the various formulations on the market today, there are some simple ideas to keep in mind when selecting the source of whey. Remember that no matter what a manufacturer might claim, there is no guarantee that your body will absorb 100 percent of the protein you ingest. Whey protein isolates contain greater than 90 percent solubility and up to 98 percent bioavailability.

As additional benefits of whey protein become clear, the popularity of this remarkable supplement will continue to grow. The fact is, for the knowledgeable athlete and health enthusiast, there is no mystery or controversy when it comes to choosing the protein source—the answer is whey. The issue then becomes one of selecting an optimal whey product.

As both a practicing physician and former champion competitive bodybuilder, I believe your choice of whey for the Greenwich Diet should be **Twinlab's Metabolift Whey Protein Meal Replacement**. The contents of this product reflect all the high points I've mentioned so far.

Metabolift Whey Protein Meal Replacement can be used two to three times each day. It comes from Twinlab, a large, well-established company. Thus, you can pretty much be assured of reliable consistency and purity. Metabolift Whey Protein Meal Replacement is fairly unique in that it contains almost no carbohydrates or fat, only pure whey protein; plus it is a convenient meal replacement providing essential vitamins and minerals. It is also rich in calcium (which is necessary when taking in large dosage amounts of protein), as well as the mineral electrolytes potassium and magnesium. This is a key point when selecting your whey protein powdered drink-mix for the Greenwich Diet.

Other reasons I favor the product include its ability to be mixed in a single serving without a blender, with only about half a cup of water. It is shocking to see how many poor quality products I've tried that are so loaded with impurities that, when added to a simple glass of water, just clump up into nauseating pasty globs. Metabolift Whey Protein Meal Replacement doesn't do that. It mixes cleanly and with little effort. And each packet is individually wrapped. Since I am always traveling about, I can't take big cans of protein with me. The small, individual packets allow me to place a couple in my briefcase, and I'm on my way.

Omega-3 Fish Oils (EPA/DHA)

As I am sure you can already tell by my bias toward the fish oils, the importance of getting the right kind of fat cannot be overemphasized. Again, as I have mentioned several times, and contrary to the popular press, your goal should not be the complete elimination of fat from the diet, but instead, elimination of the wrong kind of fat while getting more of the right kind. EPA and DHA are the right kinds of fat.

Recall that apart from the essential amino acids found in protein, fat is the only other macronutrient that has essential components. As dangerous as it is to have too much saturated fat, inadequate healthy fat in the diet will also spell disaster. The fish oil sources are the best kind of fat.

TwinEPA (from Twinlab) contains omega-3 fish oils derived from deep sea, cold-water fish. One of the attractive qualities of this particular EPA product is the fact that it offers the highest concentration and ideal combination of both EPA and DHA. Twin EPA is also the purest omega-3 fish oil product available and free of cholesterol, heavy metals and pesticides such as PCBs. In addition, this formula is fortified with additional vitamin E and fat soluble vitamin C for added antioxidant power. This product gives you a high concentration of pure n-3 fats to meet the needs of your body's essential requirements for healthy fat. In addition, by being pure n-3, TwinEPA will help offset the excess n-6 concentration that sneaks into your diet and will bring the ratio of fats into a healthy and optimum balance.

Greenwich Diet Supplement Synergy: Fat Burning in Overdrive!

There are important metabolic changes seen with excessive weight gain and obesity. Your baseline metabolism is simply a measure of how efficiently your body's engine is running. A decrease in metabolism is seen in people that gain weight or simply have excessive fat. This decrease in lean mass usually is the result of being sedentary, aging, or a combination of both. In fact, metabolic rate decreases as we age. Conventional medical theory subscribes to the notion that there is an unavoidable and irreversible loss in lean body mass and gain of fat with increasing age. Therefore, the same theorists believe we somehow require less food and nutrients. As a result, traditionalists have long suggested we need to proportionately reduce these elements. This, of course, I believe to be complete folly. So is the idea that if you are overweight or obese, you can't be malnourished. The fact is, these people need more of the essential nutrients and less non-essential, empty calories.

Just as important, as we gain fat the body's hormonal profile actually changes. From our sex hormone ratios to the levels of thyroid hormones that regulate our metabolism, excessive fat poundage throws everything out of whack. This can be extremely frustrating when dieting the conventional way because a vicious cycle ensues. When one is overweight and embarks on an intensive diet that is not properly structured or supplemented correctly, loss of any fat weight initially is all too often met with an equal slowing of metabolism. As such, leveling off when dieting can be a deeply frustrating experience that generates a tremendous dropout rate. Initially, one may need a bit more of a boost than simply dietary restriction of carbohydrates and supplementing your protein.

Apart from proper healthy Greenwich dieting, which burns a significant amount of body fat while keeping you healthy, some people might find it necessary to temporarily put fat burning into overdrive. Individuals whose metabolism has parked itself long term in the lot of sluggishness and unresponsiveness often need to jump-start their batteries, so to speak. One can do this with success using synthetic prescription stimulants (i.e., the phentermine portion of the now illegal "Phen-Fen" craze was such a stimulant). However, the use of these controlled amphetamine substances can be extremely hazardous and highly addictive.

One natural non-prescription possibility is the **Twinlab Metabolift Thermogenic Fat Burner**. This product contains both ephedrine and caffeine.

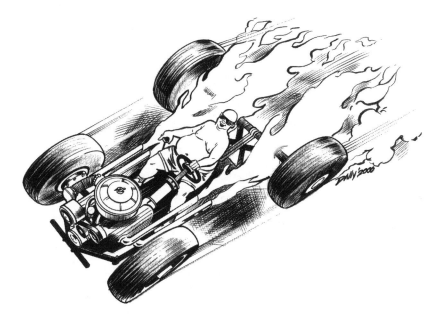

Ephedra is a natural, non-pharmaceutical stimulant available at almost any health food store. Hailing from a plant in the Pacific Rim, ephedra is a popular but controversial dietary supplement also known as Ma Huang. You might have heard of both ephedra and ephedrine. But they are not exactly synonymous. In fact, ephedra contains ephedrine. Ephedrine itself is isolated from the Ephedra sinica plant. The historical uses of ephedra have ranged from the natural treatment of wheezing and asthma, to conditions like excessive fatigue. Scientifically confirmed, this herb has become synonymous with fat burning and weight loss. In addition to the science, a large number of people report that ephedra burns fat.

Ephedra is often combined with caffeine, since caffeine has demonstrated an ability to enhance the pro-metabolic effects of ephedra. A natural source of caffeine is the guarana seed. In fact, the seed extract usually contains about 22 percent natural source caffeine.

The ephedra in the dietary capsule supplement Metabolift uses natural source Ma Huang and the caffeine comes from guarana and green tea extract. What I like about this formulation is that it contains 20 milligrams of ephedrine and 200 milligrams of caffeine per dose. These are the same amounts shown to be safe and effective for burning fat and preserving lean body mass, according to the scientific literature. Plus, the ingredients are natural and a plant source. Apart from impurities, I've always felt that natural substances are metabolized in a healthier way than many synthetics. Thus, the plant source combination of ephedra and caffeine, when taken in appropriate doses and under proper supervision, results in a metabolic lift. Subsequently, body fat is reduced.

Remember, Metabolift may put your fat burning in overdrive but you still need to be careful. Although it's natural, non-pharmaceutical and available at almost any vitamin store, you should still consult your physician before using Metabolift or any similar compound. In particular, anyone with heart problems, elevated blood pressure, or various psychological issues should especially avoid these types of substances. Beyond that, the only other concern to note is to definitely not take such substances continually. Remember, this is to be used only if you have an excessive amount of fat to lose. Other than that, you should not be taking it. Instead, better commitment to the principles of the Greenwich Diet is really the key to keeping your weight down permanently. Nonetheless, it's nice to know that there is a way to temporarily put the fat burning effect of the Greenwich Diet into overdrive.

For years both the scientific community and health enthusiasts have known about the fat burning effects of ephedrine. Ephedrine, and especially ephedrine mixed with caffeine, has been shown to be an effective aid in weight and fat loss. Unfortunately, as already mentioned, ephedrine has received some bad press because it is a stimulant substance of a higher order than caffeine. Research over the past several years has centered on searching for agents that aid in weight loss but have fewer side effects. This led to the discovery of Citrus aurantium, a natural extract isolated from fruits within the citrus family. It appears from both science and from the reports of consumers that the side effects, like those associated with ephedra consumption, are almost non-existent.

Recent research was published validating the effects of combining Citrus aurantium (six percent synephrine), caffeine and St. John's wort (**Twinlab Metabolift Ephedra-Free Thermogenic Fat Burner**) for both weight and fat loss in healthy overweight adults. The purpose of the study was to evaluate the utility in using this unique combination of ingredients for healthy weight loss as an alternative to ephedra-based products or prescription medicine. This substance falls into the class of a "thermogenic fat metabolizer and metabolic enhancer." In order to understand how this works, one must understand the thermogenic concept. Thermogenesis literally means the state of producing "new heat" within the body. You can't produce heat without burning calories—and that usually means fat loss. Compounds, like synephrine, stimulate thermogenesis by way of activating the nerve system and powering the metabolism of fat.

The synephrine contained within Citrus aurantium combined with caffeine increases the breakdown of fat and exerts mild hunger-suppressant effects. Research to date has demonstrated a metabolic enhancing quality of synephrine combined with caffeine in the form of an actual increase in the metabolic rate. In particular, synephrine/caffeine combinations may be an ideal fat burning aid for those people who have reached a plateau in their weight loss.

Studies so far have shown an increase in the metabolic rate after use of synephrine without any negative effects on blood pressure or the heart. An interesting aspect of synephrine and its parent, Citrus Aurantium, is that it is found in high amounts in orange marmalade.

The ephedra-free version of Metabolift capsules contains Citrus aurantium instead of ephedra. Like regular ephedra-containing Metabolift, ephedra-free Metabolift does contain natural caffeine from guarana and green tea extract.

In addition, ephedra-free Metabolift also contains the

natural herbal substance St. John's wort. St. John's wort is commonly known as a mild natural anti-depressant with a virtually non-existent side-effect profile. Often, when people gain excessive fat, it is from a number of factors rather than one alone. The cluster of symptoms may present itself as depression either resulting in, or resulting from, weight gain. According to the National Health and Nutrition Examination Surveys (NHANES 1-3), there is a definite correlation between depressive symptoms and weight gain. What these obesity experts found from a ten-year analysis of the NHANES data is that younger people (under 55 years) gained weight over time, while older people (over 55 years) lost weight over time and the magnitude of the weight change was greater among women at all ages. It was also established that depressive symptoms were significantly correlated with the amplification of the age-dependent weight changes.

Thus, since St. John's wort can be used to alleviate some types of mild to moderate depression, this forms the basis for its inclusion as a weight-loss adjunct in ephedra-free Metabolift. Through scientific study, this product appears to be safe and effective for short-term use in aiding fat loss and weight loss, while giving the metabolism a lift.

Nevertheless, one should still keep a few points in mind. First, like ephedra-containing Metabolift, ephedra-free Metabolift puts your fat burning in overdrive but without some of the risks associated with ephedra. Even so, you need to be careful. Although ephedra-free Metabolift contains Citrus aurantium (synephrine containing) instead of the Ma Huang found in ephedra-containing Metabolift, I still believe you need to exert the same caution. It is a widely held belief that, unlike ephedra, synephrine should not increase heart rate and blood pressure. Still, it is advisable to consult your physician first. Beyond that, the same rules apply in terms of not taking this substance continually. As with ephedra-containing Metabolift, ephedra-free Metabolift should only be used if you have an excessive amount of weight to lose. Again, commitment to the principles of the Greenwich Diet is the key to keeping your weight down permanently. Even so, it's nice to know there is an ephedra-free alternative to Metabolift and another way to temporarily put the fat burning effect of the Greenwich Diet into overdrive.

$\mathcal{A}$ SIMPLE UNDERSTANDING
of the GREENWICH DIET
VII

Fundamentals of the Greenwich Diet

Basic Guidelines, Rules, and Principles at a Glance

Macronutrient Overview

Carbohydrates:

1. 30-100 grams of carbohydrates for non-exercisers, 50-200 grams of carbohydrates for exercisers. If you are used to taking in a lot of carbohydrates, work this level down gradually and pay attention to your body because too drastic a drop is uncomfortable, not to mention unmanageable.

2. With the exception of what might be contained in one of your dietary supplements, incidental carbohydrates only (i.e., your only source of sugar should be from the carbohydrates that happen to occur in relatively small amounts within fibrous vegetables); no carbohydrate based foods.

3. No starchy foods (rice, pasta, white bread, potatoes, corn, etc.). Learn the difference between a carbohydrate-based vegetable like corn or yams and a fiber-based vegetable like lettuce or celery. Although bread is not part of the Greenwich Diet, if you are tempted on rare occasion, a heavy whole grain bread only in moderation and in the morning or mid-afternoon isn't such a terrible thing.

4. Avoid fruits. Don't kid yourself, they're simple sugars. If you feel you need one once in a while, choose apples because of their relatively high fiber and pectin content.

5. At least in the beginning, while building up your fiber intake, be sure to take a good daily multivitamin/multimineral supplement so your body isn't missing any of these elements.

Protein:

1. Predominantly whey protein, but also whole eggs or egg whites, skim milk, lean steak, chicken breast and fish.

2. Absolutely no ham, bacon, or other pork products (nitrates and nitrites).

3. Absolutely no soy or soy products.

4. 50 percent of all protein should consist of whey protein (such as Twinlab's Metablolift Whey Protein Meal Replacement). This makes meals small and extremely convenient.

5. Minimum protein intake of 0.8 grams per pound of body

weight for non-exercisers, with at least 1.3 grams per pound of body weight for heavy exercisers.
6. Protein meals should consist of between 25 and 30 grams per feeding.
7. Protein meals should be spaced throughout the day by 2.0 to 3.0 hours for non-exercisers and up to 1.5 to 2.0 hours for heavy exercisers.

Fat:

1. Limit an excess of "direct" animal fat (butter, cream, lard, cheese, fatty meat).
2. "Indirect" animal fat sources that have a low incidental fat content are permissible (fish, chicken, eggs, lean steak, rabbit, game, etc.).
3. Of the vegetable oils, avoid corn, safflower and sunflower oil.
4. 1,000 to 2,000 milligrams per day of EPA/DHA (Twinlab TwinEPA) supplementation for non-exercisers; 1,500 to 3,000 milligrams per day of EPA/DHA gel-cap supplementation for heavy exercisers
5. Olive oil should be added to the diet for cooking and for salads.

Fiber:

• A lot of high fiber, non-starch vegetables (lettuce, peppers, asparagus, cabbage, Brussels sprouts, broccoli, cau-

liflower, carrots, onions, spinach, etc.). Five to seven servings of fiber per day should be adequate. (A serving is
between four and six grams).

Water:

• Minimum of one gallon of water (16 glasses) each day
for exercisers; minimum one-half gallon (eight glasses) each
day for non-exercisers.

Basic Concepts

The Greenwich Diet is a meal plan designed to induce a
special type of metabolism that actually reduces physical
hunger after 72 hours of adjustment. Do your best to stick
with the plan during the toughest time, which is just in the
beginning. After that, it gets incredibly easy. But be careful,
deviations from this diet early on will make the plan less
successful. You may initially crave starchy carbohydrates
(rice, bread, potatoes, pasta, sugar products) but this
craving will rapidly diminish after the first few days.
Remember, if you are used to consuming a lot of
carbohydrates, you may have to reduce them gradually
depending on how you feel.

The great advantage of the Greenwich Diet is that you
will eat frequently throughout the day while actually losing
weight and burning fat off your body.

General Principles

- Meals should be spaced about every 1-1/2 to 2-1/2 hours apart. To accomplish this, we incorporate a snack between breakfast-lunch and lunch-dinner. Remember, when following the Greenwich Diet, snacks count as meals. So, you will actually end up having about five to six meals a day, yet still lose weight!
- Avoid eating after dinner.
- Foods high in carbohydrates are the enemy. Keep to an absolute minimum all carbohydrate-rich foods such as cookies, candies, cakes, pies and even fruit, dried fruit, fruit juices, rice, pasta, bread, potatoes, and corn. If you have to have a fruit, go with apples because of their relatively high fiber content.
- Foods high in dietary fiber and relatively low in carbohydrates are friends. Trace carbohydrates found in high fiber vegetables are fine (i.e., celery, lettuce, cucumber, spinach, carrots, etc...).
- Make sure to include two to three servings of Twinlab Metabolift Whey Protein Meal Replacement in addition to your protein food.
- Avoid ham, bacon and pork products.
- Nothing beats fish containing EPA/DHA. Eating cold-water fish is great and highly encouraged in the Greenwich Diet, but you will invariably need to supplement with omega-3 fish oils.
- Avoid an excess of unhealthy animal fats such as butter, cream and lard. Not all vegetable oil is healthy either. Remember, corn oil is a disaster. Olive oil is best.

• Make sure to drink plenty of water—one gallon (16 glasses) per day for exercisers and one-half gallon (eight glasses) per day for non-exercisers.

Exercise and the Greenwich Diet

Exercise and nutrition are indisputably linked. No matter how effective any diet might be in the short term, you can't expect lasting results without combining it with exercise. It's like trying to drive a car across town while running on fumes. For a little while everything is going to work and seem okay. But soon, the car will sputter and grind to a halt. Don't let anyone kid you, exercise is an integral part of healthy living and subsequently must be part of your life.

Exercise provides many benefits that complement the Greenwich Diet. Regular exercise can lower your risk of heart disease, high blood pressure and high cholesterol. Increasing physical activity can lower harmful triglycerides and raise the good form of cholesterol called HDL. Physical activity also protects against development of breast cancer and osteoporosis in women. Exercise can prevent strokes as well as restore function following a stroke. Being more physically active will prevent or delay vascular complications associated with diabetes and may also reduce the need for insulin. A well-designed exercise program enhances joint stability and prevents, lessens, or even reverses the bone loss seen in aging. Exercise can help reduce symptoms of depression and anxiety while increasing energy levels and preventing obesity.

Although I always tell my clients and patients that cardiovascular training and recreational sports are terrific, I lean toward a more structured approach. The reason for this preference is that I don't want those I care for to confuse activity and exercise. The word "exercise" is relative. For example, when a 50-year-old woman has worked all day in her garden, despite her exhaustion at the end of the day, she did not exercise. Although quite active, her experience gardening does not constitute exercise. Similarly, a 45-year-old man walking around all day at the mall with his family may be extremely fatigued at day's end, but he didn't exercise either.

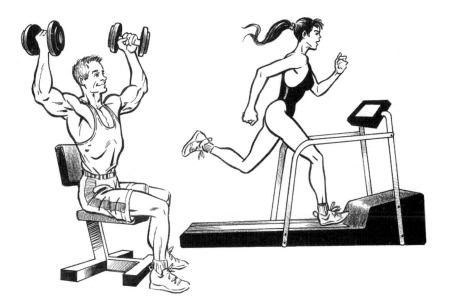

Unlike exhaustive activity, which may very well be health beneficial at a certain level, exercise is a focused, proactive challenging of the body's limits. True exercise is more intense than simple activity. But again, exercise is relative. When my 97-year-old patient is able to make her way around the block without the use of her walker, it is a short-term accomplishment for which she must exert tremendous effort. When she does this, I consider it exercise. I certainly wouldn't consider a walk around the block exercise for a healthy 40-year-old man. Unfortunately, society has become so lazy that too many 40-year-old men confuse the activity of walking around the block with exercise.

Exercise, to me, means exerting oneself for a specific purpose and with focused intensity. By creating structured sessions of exercise you will not have to rely on a potential misperception of whether or not you are exercising or just being active. Also, only by setting aside a definite time for exercise do you actually begin to learn something about yourself. Since a primary goal of the Greenwich Diet is to teach you something about yourself, it makes sense to incorporate exercise. The two approaches complement each other.

Exercise should be done at least three days per week for 20 minutes or more. Remember, these should be focused sessions of challenging physical exertion, so walking the dog doesn't count as exercise, but rather as activity. Most exercises fall into one of two categories—aerobic or cardiovascular exercise and anaerobic or resistive exercise. Aerobic activity is not just beneficial for esthetic reasons such as toning and weight loss, but such cardiovascular training reduces the risk of heart disease and stroke, while decreasing blood pressure and high cholesterol. Aerobic training has even been shown to help in everything from improving your immune status to reducing symptoms of PMS (great news for both men and women!).

Typical aerobic work should be done on cardiovascular equipment including bikes, treadmills, cross-trainers and stair climbers. As a general rule I tend to stay away from running unless it involves sprinting or running up a hill or stairs. This is because the injury potential is so dramatically high in traditional flat surface running. Also, most people who think they are running are, in fact, walking fast and, at best, jogging or trotting along at a relatively unchallenging pace. What ends up happening is that they invest far too much time in this mind and body-numbing experience, sometimes to the tune of hours each day. In my experience, far greater cardiovascular and metabolic stimulation is achieved by challenging your age-predicted heart rate maximum and VO2 max as we physicians do in a stress test. This means working at a higher intensity for a shorter duration. Forget about counting calories burned and leave that to the Greenwich Diet. Concentrate more on increasing your intensity to stimulate your metabolism.

In order for each training bout to be effective, you should first properly calculate your training heart rate range. To do so, obtain an accurate resting heart rate by measuring your pulse when you first wake up in the morning. Use this number to calculate your target heart rate range. This range can be calculated using Karvonen's Formula, as follows:

(220-Age) – (Resting Heart Rate) x (0.6) + Resting Heart Rate = Rate #1

(220-Age) – (Resting Heart Rate) x (0.8) + Resting Heart Rate = Rate #2

These two numbers will give you 60 to 80 percent of your heart rate range. When exercising for your cardiovascular fitness, make it a point to stay within the upper range of these two numbers. Attempting to maintain this heart rate will be challenging. In fact, most people that do a mind and body numbing jog are not conscious of these numbers and are therefore never really working hard enough to benefit themselves significantly. Of course, exercising in such a way from a cardiovascular standpoint is quite a bit more challenging than traditional jogging, so make sure your own physician gives you a clean bill of health and that you start slowly and work your way up. Five minutes of such intense work is terrific. If you can work up to twenty minutes, you must increase the level of difficulty (i.e., steeper incline on a treadmill or greater resistance on a bike, for example). My personal favorite is stair climbing. It is significantly difficult that I am able to challenge my predicted maximum heart rate while keeping my total time spent doing cardio-training to an efficient minimum.

Either way, although more difficult, your sessions will be much shorter and less time consuming than traditional jogging. In addition, they will be more beneficial. People who jog for hours probably do so out of some obsessive behavior coupled with the misguided notion that more running means more calorie burning. Sadly, most such individuals jog for hours but never get their diets straight. Think about how many people you see jogging for hours who have an excessive amount of fat on their bodies that they claim they've never been able to lose. The problem is that they don't apply the fundamentals of good eating into this model. Those on the Greenwich Diet never have to rely on exercise to "burn calories." The diet takes care of that issue. As a result, you can naturally shorten the monotonous duration of traditional cardiovascular exercise, turn up the intensity, and really get the benefits you are supposed to receive from aerobic work.

Of equal importance is the anaerobic or resistive form of exercise. Resistive training primarily means weight training, but also includes calisthenics. Resistive training is a significant component of physical fitness and, like cardiovascular training, complements the Greenwich Diet. Resistive training offers the benefits of increased strength and higher bone density. Such forms of exercise have been shown to positively influence the body's hormonal system. Resistive exercise also creates more lean muscle, which makes it easier to lose body fat. Resistive training is more compatible with activities of daily living and thus can dramatically enhance the quality and ease of one's life. Resistive training also builds physical confidence in one's body. In addition, there is mounting evidence that resistive training bolsters the immune system and strengthens the body's internal fortitude in both men and women.

Using weights to train is probably the single greatest resistive workout you can do to benefit your health. People are generally smart and know a good thing when they see it. Anyone who ever trains with weights for any reasonable length of time quickly recognizes the benefits. Their bodies not only look better, but feel better and stronger. Clearly, weight training for people young and old has literally swept the nation. In fact, as an individual with a brutal travel schedule, I can tell you first hand that almost everywhere I go, even the smallest towns in America, I can invariably find some kind of weight training facility.

Weight training typically involves either free weights or machine weights. For beginners, those with injuries, or individuals with physical limitations, machines are ideal to start with. The weight is already in the "down position" prior to exerting force. The "stack" is balanced and tressled for you, lending control to the motion throughout its course. Just remember that if it's not a physical limitation that is hindering you, these same benefits ultimately prove to be the limiting factor. With free weights you must control the bar, balance the weight and move it smoothly through a given range of motion. For these reasons, free weights require the incorporation and recruitment of far deeper muscle fibers. This is a much taller order than working on a machine. It is for these reasons that free weight exercises tend to ultimately be more beneficial for both men and women. But free weight training, unlike machines, is really an art form and getting some instruction is usually your best bet. A good personal trainer can start you on machine weights and then gradually incorporate more free-weight motions to the point that free weight training becomes the predominant resistive work you are doing, with machine weights only part of your routine as an adjunct. But even if you are training alone, although machine weights represent a great place to start because they are easy to figure out, beyond the beginning stages of training there should be a gradual progression and, ultimately, a clear preference toward free weights.

Beyond cardiovascular work and resistive training, there are other elements to fitness and total body health that complement the Greenwich Diet and should not be ignored. Flexibility and stretching are extremely important because quite a number of injuries can be traced to poor flexibility and limited range of motion. In general, flexibility and functionality go hand-in-hand. You don't have to overdo it, since just a little stretching after your workouts is all it takes to maximize the benefits of exercise and minimize the likelihood of injury.

I'm also a great believer in proper healthy breathing. As a former power lifter, I have always traced my strength to my breathing pattern. Later on, as a physician and as a result of my experience, I began to take note of the way my patients were breathing. In particular, my sicker hospitalized patients tended to take shallow, quick breaths through their noses with lips pursed. I also began noticing this pattern had less to do with the type of illness the patient suffered from and more to do with the degree of seriousness of the illness, with the worst patterns being demonstrated in the intensive care unit. Interestingly, as the patients' conditions would improve, their breathing would become slower and deeper. Their faces were more relaxed and they tended to draw more air through their mouths. Back then, I was somewhat certain this breathing pattern was a result of illness. However, later on in my practice, with more experience in a non-disease-based, clinical wellness setting, I began realizing that there was a definite cause and effect. Subsequently, I have come to the firm conclusion that deep, slow breathing is synonymous with good health. Of great reassurance to me was a lecture I attended by Andrew Weil, M.D. He spoke at great length about the healthy power of breathing. Perhaps the ancient grand practitioners of yoga were right and Dr. Weil and I have done nothing more than come upon a long forgotten precious gem of knowledge.

With all this in mind, I should emphasize that the best place to learn about proper healthy breathing is to exercise. When you begin to exercise, you suddenly become very conscious of your breathing. The depth of your breath, the rapidity, the quality, and the mechanism all begin to speak to you. Don't panic and don't ignore your breathing. Bathe in the quality of air moving throughout your body and appreciate the newfound chorus that is speaking to you, for it is a key to health and wellness and in keeping with the Greenwich Diet.

GETTING STARTED *on the* GREENWICH DIET

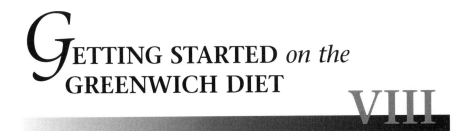

VIII

Sample Programs and Sample 7-Day Diet Plan

The sample programs and diet plans that follow are merely general examples of actual applications of the Greenwich Diet and may not necessarily apply to you. For example, although I differentiate between programs for exercisers and non-exercisers (of course, preferring that you exercise) in terms of maintenance versus fat burning, there are still an infinite number of variations of individual preference. In other words, a 250-pound male might need considerably larger serving sizes than the smaller serving sizes appropriate for a 135-pound female. Nonetheless, the food choices and nutrient categories are the same. Remember that the Greenwich Diet is not based on calorie counting, percentages of macronutrients, or ratios of foods to one another. Instead, the Greenwich Diet is a healthy eating plan for low body fat and high energy levels.

Non-Exerciser's Sample Maintenance Program

MEAL COLUMN	SNACK COLUMN

Breakfast
2 Twinlab Metabolift multivitamins, 1-3 TwinEPA gelcaps to
be taken with breakfast, at
least 2 glasses of water

Egg omelet made with 2-3 eggs
1 cup steamed vegetables
1 Tbs. Parmesan cheese or salsa
Coffee, tea or bottled water

Mid-Morning Protein Snack
1 Twinlab Metabolift Whey Protein
Meal Replacement Drink or choose
one of the following & include at
least 1 glass of water:

- 1 hard boiled egg
- 3/4 cup low-fat cottage cheese
- 1 cup sugar-free Dannon®
  Light yogurt

Lunch
2 glasses of water with lunch

4-6 oz. lean meat/fish/poultry/
seafood (no ham or pork)
2 cups steamed vegetables
2 cups mixed green salad
(use balsamic vinegar
& olive oil)

Mid-Afternoon Snack
1 Twinlab Metabolift Whey Protein
Meal Replacement Drink or choose
one of the following & include at
least 1 glass of water:

- 1 hard boiled egg
- 3/4 cup low-fat cottage cheese
- 1 cup sugar-free Dannon®
  Light yogurt

Dinner
1-3 TwinEPA gelcaps to be taken
with dinner, 2 glasses of water
with dinner &

2-3 cups mixed green salad
(use balsamic vinegar &
olive oil)
4-6 oz. lean meat/fish/
poultry/seafood
(no ham or pork)
2 cups steamed vegetables

After Dinner Snack
Choose one of the following:

- 1 Twinlab Metabolift Whey
  Protein Meal Replacement
  Drink
- 1 cup vegetable sticks

*No eating following after-dinner
snack.*

Exerciser's Sample Maintenance Program

MEAL COLUMN	SNACK COLUMN

MEAL COLUMN

Breakfast
2 Twinlab Metabolift multivitamins, 2-4 TwinEPA gelcaps to
be taken with breakfast, at
least 2 glasses of water

Egg omelet made with 2-3 eggs
1 cup steamed vegetables
1 Tbs. Parmesan cheese or salsa

Lunch
2 glasses of water with lunch

4-6 oz. lean meat/fish/poultry/
seafood (no ham or pork)
2 cups steamed vegetables
2 cups mixed green salad
(use balsamic vinegar &
olive oil)

Dinner
1-3 TwinEPA gelcaps to be taken
with dinner
2 glasses of water with dinner

2-3 cups mixed green salad
(use balsamic vinegar &
olive oil)
4-6 oz. lean meat/fish/poultry/
seafood (no ham or pork)
2 cups steamed vegetables

SNACK COLUMN

Mid-Morning Protein Snack
1 Twinlab Metabolift Whey
Protein Meal Replacement
Drink or choose one of the
following & include at least 1
glass of water:

- 1 hard boiled egg
- 3/4 cup low-fat cottage cheese
- 1 cup sugar-free Dannon®
Light yogurt

Mid-Afternoon Snack
1 Twinlab Metabolift Whey
Protein Meal Replacement
Drink or choose one of the
following & include at least 1
glass of water:

- 1 hard boiled egg
- 3/4 cup low-fat cottage cheese
- 1 cup sugar-free Dannon®
Light yogurt

Late-Afternoon Snack
1 Twinlab Metabolift Whey
Protein Meal Replacement
Drink or 1 cup low-fat cottage
cheese

After Dinner Snack
Choose one of the following:

- 1 Twinlab Metabolift Whey
Protein Meal Replacement
Drink
- 1 cup vegetable sticks

*No eating following after-dinner
snack.*

Non-Exerciser's Sample Fat Burning Program

MEAL COLUMN	SNACK COLUMN

Breakfast
  2 Twinlab Metabolift multivitamins, 1-3 TwinEPA gelcaps to
  be taken with breakfast, 1-2
  Metabolift capsules (ephedra
  or ephedra free), at least 2
  glasses of water

Egg omelet made with 2-3 eggs
1 cup steamed vegetables
1 Tbs. Parmesan cheese or salsa

Mid-Morning Protein Snack
  1 Twinlab Metabolift Whey
  Protein Meal Replacement
  Drink or 2 hard boiled eggs

Lunch
  8-ounce glass of water
  with lunch,
  1-2 Twinlab Metabolift capsules
  (ephedra or ephedra free)

4-6 oz. lean meat/fish/poultry/
  seafood (no ham or pork)
2 cups steamed vegetables
2 cups mixed green salad
  (use balsamic vinegar &
  olive oil)

Mid-Afternoon Snack
  1 Twinlab Metabolift Whey
  Protein Meal Replacement
  Drink.
  Add at least 1 glass of water

Dinner
  1-3 TwinEPA gelcaps to be taken
  with dinner
2 glasses of water with dinner

2-3 cups mixed green salad
  (use balsamic vinegar &
  olive oil)
4-6 oz. lean meat/fish/poultry/
  seafood (no ham or pork)
2 cups steamed vegetables

Exerciser Sample Fat Burning Program

MEAL COLUMN	SNACK COLUMN

MEAL COLUMN

Breakfast
2 Twinlab Metabolift multivitamins, 2-4 TwinEPA gelcaps to
   be taken with breakfast, 1-2
   Metabolift capsules (ephedra
   or ephedra free), at least 2
   glasses of water

Egg omelet made with 2-3 eggs
1 cup steamed vegetables
1 Tbs. Parmesan cheese or salsa

Lunch
1-2 Twinlab Metabolift capsules
   (ephedra or ephedra free)
2 glasses of water with lunch

4-6 oz. lean meat/fish/poultry/
   seafood (no ham or pork)
2 cups steamed vegetables
2 cups mixed green salad
(use balsamic vinegar &
   olive oil)

Dinner
4-8 TwinEPA gelcaps to be taken
   with dinner
2 glasses of water with dinner
2-3 cups mixed green salad
(use balsamic vinegar &
   olive oil)
4-6 oz. lean meat/fish/poultry/
   seafood (no ham or pork)
2 cups steamed vegetables

SNACK COLUMN

Mid-Morning Protein Snack
1 Twinlab Metabolift Whey
   Protein Meal Replacement
   Drink or choose one of the
   following & include at least 1
   glass of water:

• 1 hard boiled egg
• 3/4 cup low-fat cottage cheese
• 1 cup sugar-free Dannon®
   Light yogurt

Mid-Afternoon Snack
1 Twinlab Metabolift Whey
   Protein Meal Replacement
   Drink or choose one of the
   following & include at least 1
   glass of water:

• 1 hard boiled egg
• 3/4 cup low-fat cottage cheese
• 1 cup sugar-free Dannon®
   Light yogurt

Late-Afternoon Snack
• 1 Twinlab Metabolift Whey
   Protein Meal Replacement
   Drink or 1 cup low-fat cottage
   cheese

No eating following after-dinner snack

Sample 7 Day Diet Plan

Day 1

MEAL COLUMN	SNACK COLUMN

Breakfast–8am
- 8oz. coffee or tea or water
- 2 Twinlab Metabolift multivitamins
- 2 TwinEPA gelcaps
- 1 Twinlab Metabolift Whey Protein Meal Replacement Drink
- 1 Cup of sugar free Dannon® Light Yogurt

Mid-Morning Protein Snack–10am
- 8 oz. sugar-free Dannon® Light yogurt
- 8 oz. water (additionally)

Lunch–12 noon
- 6 oz. tuna fish
- 2 cups mixed green salad w/balsamic vinegar and olive oil
- 8 oz. water

Mid-Afternoon Snack–2pm
- 1 Twinlab Metabolift Whey Protein Meal Replacement or 2 slices of turkey breast

Late-Afternoon Snack–4pm
- 1 Twinlab Metabolift Whey Protein Meal Replacement or 2 slices of turkey breast

Dinner–6pm
- 2 cups mixed green salad w/2 Tbs. balsamic vinegar and olive oil
- 5 oz. filet mignon
- 1.5 cups steamed broccoli w/2 Tbs. grated cheese
- 2 TwinEPA gelcaps

After Dinner Snack–8pm
- 1 Twinlab Metabolift Whey Protein Meal Replacement or 2 hard boiled eggs

Day 2

MEAL COLUMN	SNACK COLUMN

Breakfast–8am
2 eggs low-fat cheese omelet
  with salsa to taste
8 oz. coffee or tea or water
2 Twinlab Metabolift
  multivitamin
2 TwinEPA gelcaps

Mid-Morning Protein Snack–10am
1 Twinlab Metabolift Whey
  Protein Meal Replacement
  Drink
8 oz. water (additionally)

Lunch–12 noon
1/4 pound lean roast beef
2 cups steamed cauliflower
  w/virgin olive oil, lemon and
  spices to taste
8 oz. water

Mid-Afternoon Snack–2pm
1 Twinlab Metabolift Whey
  Protein Meal Replacement
  Drink or 2 slices turkey breast
1 medium carrot

Dinner–6pm
2 cups mixed green and tomato
  salad
w/balsamic vinegar and olive oil
8 oz. broiled salmon w/dill,
  lemon and mustard
2 cups steamed green beans
  w/olive oil, pepper and garlic
2 TwinEPA gelcaps

Late-Afternoon Snack–4pm
1 Twinlab Metabolift Whey
  Protein Meal Replacement
  Drink

After Dinner Snack–8pm
1 cup vegetable sticks (carrots
  &/or celery mix)

Day 3

MEAL COLUMN	SNACK COLUMN

Breakfast–8am
- 2-3 egg vegetable omelet
- 8 oz. coffee or tea
- 2 Twinlab Metabolift multivitamins
- 2 TwinEPA gelcaps

Mid-Morning Protein Snack–10am
- 1 Twinlab Metabolift Whey Protein Meal Replacement Drink
- 8 oz. water (additionally)

Lunch–12 noon
- Canned white albacore tuna w/3 Tbs. balsamic vinegar
- 1 cup lettuce, peppers, onions and mushrooms salad
- 2 oz. turkey breast

Mid-Afternoon Snack–2pm
- 1 Twinlab Metabolift Whey Protein Meal Replacement Drink

Late-Afternoon Snack–4pm
- 8 oz. sugar-free Dannon Light® yogurt
- 8 oz. water

Dinner–6pm
- 2 cups mixed green salad w/balsamic vinegar and olive oil
- 8 oz. "Olive Stuffed Flounder" - see recipe
- 1 cup boiled asparagus w/virgin olive oil and salted to taste
- 12 oz. water
- 2 TwinEPA gelcaps

After Dinner Snack–8pm
- 1 Twinlab Metabolift Whey Protein Meal Replacement Drink or 2 hard boiled eggs

Day 4

MEAL COLUMN	SNACK COLUMN

Breakfast–8am
- 1 serving of "Spinach and Feta Omelet" - see recipe
- 8 oz. coffee or tea or water
- 2 Twinlab Metabolift multivitamins
- 2 TwinEPA gelcaps

Mid-Morning Protein Snack–10am
- 1 Twinlab Metabolift Whey Protein Meal Replacement Drink
- 8 oz. water (additionally)

Lunch–12 noon
- 1 serving "Monaco Salad" - see recipe
- w/2 Tbs. salad dressing
- 6 oz. grilled chicken breast
- 8 oz. water

Mid-Afternoon Snack–2pm
- 8 oz. sugar-free Dannon® light yogurt (any flavor)
- 1 hard-boiled egg
- 8oz. water

Late-Afternoon Snack–4pm
- 1 Twinlab Metabolift Whey Protein Meal Replacement Drink or 3 slices turkey breast

Dinner–6pm
- 6oz. "Sherried Mushroom Chicken" - see recipe
- 1 cup cooked spinach
- 8 oz. Diet Coke® soda or Diet Snapple® iced-tea
- 8 oz. water
- 2 TwinEPA gelcaps

After Dinner Snack–8pm
- 1 Twinlab Metabolift Whey Protein Meal Replacement Drink
- 8oz. water (additionally)

Day 5

MEAL COLUMN	SNACK COLUMN

Breakfast–8am
1 cup low-fat cottage cheese
8oz. coffee, tea, or water
2 Twinlab Metabolift
multivitamins
2 TwinEPA gelcaps

Mid-Morning Protein Snack–10am
1 Twinlab Metabolift Whey
Protein Meal Replacement
Drink or 2 hard boiled eggs

Lunch–12 noon
6oz. turkey burger (without bun)
1 cup raw carrot sticks
12 oz. Diet Coke® soda or water

Mid-Afternoon Snack–2pm
1 Twinlab Metabolift Whey
Protein Meal Replacement
Drink or 1 cup low-fat cottage
cheese

Dinner–6pm
1 serving of "Tangy Salsa Red
Snapper" - see recipe
1 cup broccoli sautéed in 1Tbs.
olive oil and 1 garlic clove
12 oz. Diet Snapple® iced tea or
flavored seltzer water
2 TwinEPA gelcaps

Late-Afternoon Snack–4pm
1 cup sugar-free Dannon® light
yogurt

After Dinner Snack–8pm
1 Twinlab Metabolift Whey
Protein Meal Replacement
Drink
8 oz. water (additionally)

Day 6

MEAL COLUMN	SNACK COLUMN

Breakfast–8am
3 scrambled eggs
w/stir fried peppers and onions
2 Twinlab Metabolift
   multivitamins
2 TwinEPA gelcaps

Mid-Morning Protein Snack–10am
1 Twinlab Metabolift Whey
Protein Meal Replacement
Drink
8 oz. water (additionally) or
1 cup low-fat cottage cheese

Lunch–12 noon
Shrimp salad made with
2 cups green salad
1.5 cups chopped cucumbers
6 oz. grilled shrimp
12 oz. water

Mid-Afternoon Snack–2pm
1 Twinlab Metabolift Whey
Protein Meal Replacement
Drink
8 oz. water (additionally)

Late-Afternoon Snack–4pm
1 Twinlab Metabolift Whey
Protein Meal Replacement
Drink or 3 slices turkey breast

Dinner–6pm
2 cups mixed green salad
w/balsamic vinegar and olive oil
6 oz. broiled swordfish w/garlic,
   black pepper and olive oil
4 items of "Spinach Stuffed
   Mushrooms" - see recipe
12 oz. water
2 TwinEPA gelcaps

After Dinner Snack–8pm
1 Twinlab Metabolift Whey
Protein Meal Replacement
Drink

Day 7

MEAL COLUMN	SNACK COLUMN

MEAL COLUMN

Breakfast–8am
8 oz. sugar-free Dannon® light
  yogurt
12 oz. water
2 Twinlab Metabolift
  multivitamins
2 TwinEPA gelcaps

Lunch–12 noon
1/4 pound of sliced chicken
  breast
2 cups mixed green salad
w/balsamic vinegar and olive oil
8 oz. Diet Coke® soda, Diet
  Snapple® iced tea, or water

Dinner–6pm
2 cups spinach and
  romaine salad
w/balsamic vinegar and olive oil
Steak and Vegetable Stir Fry
w/ 2Tbs. olive oil:
6 oz. lean red meat (cubed)
1 cup snow peas
1/2 cup onions
  Add soy sauce/teriyaki sauce
  for taste
12oz. flavored seltzer water or
  regular water
2 TwinEPA gelcaps

SNACK COLUMN

Mid-Morning Protein Snack–10am
1 Twinlab Metabolift Whey
  Protein Meal Replacement
  Drink or 2 hard boiled eggs

Mid-Afternoon Snack–2pm
1 Twinlab Metabolift Whey
  Protein Meal Replacement
  Drink
8oz. water (additionally)

Late-Afternoon Snack–4pm
3/4 cup low-fat cottage cheese
8 oz. water

After Dinner Snack–8pm
1 Twinlab Metabolift Whey
  Protein Meal Replacement
  Drink or 1 cup low-fat cottage
  cheese

Shopping & Food Labels

Greenwich Diet Shopping List

Fluids:
- [ ] Water
- [ ] Seltzer water (flavored or unflavored)
- [ ] Diet Coke® soda
- [ ] Coffee
- [ ] Tea (hot or cold)

Protein:
- [ ] *Whey protein
- [ ] Fish (cold water fish like salmon, tuna, mackerel and herring are best) and other seafood including swordfish, lobster, and shrimp are fine as well.
- [ ] Low-fat cheese
- [ ] Eggs or egg whites
- [ ] Lean steak and all other lean red meat including filet mignon, rib rye, shell, strip, porterhouse, sirloin, London broil, as well as high-quality ground beef are excellent choices.
- [ ] Veal
- [ ] Lamb
- [ ] Chicken breast and turkey
- [ ] Sugar-free yogurt
- [ ] Low-fat cottage cheese

*Available at your vitamin or health food store

Fats & Oils:
- [ ] Olive oil
- [ ] *EPA/DHA – omega-3 fish oils
- [ ] Flaxseed oil

Sources of Fiber:
- [ ] Artichokes
- [ ] Asparagus
- [ ] Avocado
- [ ] Beets
- [ ] Broccoli
- [ ] Brussels sprouts
- [ ] Cabbage
- [ ] Carrots
- [ ] Cauliflower
- [ ] Celery
- [ ] Collard greens
- [ ] Cucumber
- [ ] Eggplant
- [ ] Kale
- [ ] Lettuce – (romaine is far superior to iceberg in fiber content)
- [ ] Mushrooms
- [ ] Okra
- [ ] Onions
- [ ] Peppers
- [ ] Radishes
- [ ] Snow peas
- [ ] Spinach
- [ ] Squash
- [ ] String beans
- [ ] Swiss chard

Understanding Food Label Information

Don't be fooled by a clever play on words used by a product manufacturer. Understanding the meaning of food labeling can almost be an art! The definitions that follow will help you understand exactly what it is you are buying and whether those products are consistent with the Greenwich Diet.

"Free"
The food contains only a tiny amount of fat, sugar, cholesterol or sodium. For example, a food labeled "fat-free" contains less than 0.5 grams of fat per serving.

"Low"
Food labeled "low-fat" contains no more than 3 grams of fat per serving.

"Lean" and "Extra Lean"
USDA terms for meat and poultry. "Lean" means the meat contains less than 10 grams of fat per 3.5 ounce serving. "Extra lean" means the meat contains less than 5 grams of fat per 3.5 ounce serving.

"Reduced," "Less" or "Fewer"
These words mean that the food has 1/4 less of a nutrient or calories. For example, hot dogs containing 25% less fat than regular hot dogs could be labeled "reduced-fat" or "25% less fat."

"Light" or "Lite"

This means the food has a 1/2 less of a nutrient, or 1/3 fewer calories than the original food. For example, a food labeled "lite cheddar cheese" contains 1/2 the fat of regular cheddar cheese.

"More"

This means that one serving of the food contains at least 10% more of the daily value of a vitamin, mineral or fiber than usual.

"Good source of"

This means that one serving of the food contains 10-19% of the daily value for a particular vitamin, mineral or fiber.

Dining In & Dining Out for the Greenwich Dieter

Dining In on the Greenwich Diet

Cooking Tips

It has been my belief for many years that the longer you cook something, the more unhealthy it becomes. Healthy food simply doesn't need to be cooked that long. With increased cooking time, vital nutrients are leeched out and lost to oblivion. With further exposure, fiber loses its roughage. Still further, burnt or blackened food is a sure cancer-causing carcinogen.

Although I like my burgers medium-rare, the meat I make them from is of high quality. Overcooking any red meat destroys nutrients and flavor. However, if the quality of your meat is poor (the kind I suggest avoiding), over-cooking can save your life. In fact, did you ever see those warnings on the news about fast food hamburgers not being cooked enough? As a result, people periodically get violently ill and even die from E. coli (a bacteria) exposure. The recommendation to the public as a result of these out-breaks is always to make sure we get our burgers well cooked! How disgusting! To my recollection, not a single news source has told us not to eat this garbage. I urge you to avoid fast-food red meat.

Perhaps this best describes why I have a ban on pork and pork products for my Greenwich Dieters. Apart from the cancer-causing nitrites and/or smoking process, the incredibly high saturated fat content, and the loads of sodium, there is something unique to pig meat, and innate-ly grotesque. Jews and Muslims have held to the belief for thousands of years that the pig is unclean and not for human consumption. Are they all just crazy? I don't think so. Perhaps there is something to be learned from this belief. But, if you can't take their word for it, science tells us that the parasite *Trichinella spiralis* (a parasitic worm) liter-ally lives in pork meat. The worm is a regular inhabitant of pork meat. In fact, infestation is so common and wide-spread that I recall as far back as my high school science class taking a piece of bacon and looking at the encrusted larva under a microscope. This isn't like a simple bacteria that once in a while can be found in food (like occasional salmonella in chicken). No. Quite the contrary. This is an animal. A worm. A multicellular parasite that loves pig flesh. Humans can be infected from poorly cooked pork. The symptoms are harsh, painful and may even be deadly. As a physician I can tell you there is no specific treatment. In fairness to pigs, there aren't many cases in America because most people that eat pork cook it pretty well, but then you are back to my theory on overcooking being innately nutrient-poor and unhealthy. Bottom line—even though cooking kills the parasite, you still have to eat the dead parasitic worm in the pig flesh. Sorry to be so graphic, but hopefully that convinces you to take a pass on pork.

Back to cooking tips! Deep-frying is a big fat crime. Boiling won't expose you to the fat and lard, but too long of a boil and you'll be left with some kind of food product bereft of any nutrient content because it escapes into the liquid. If you want to cook this way and still get all the nutrients, be sure and drink the water after you choke down that "misery biscuit" you're mistaking for food.

In general, the healthier preference is to steam or broil food. However, stir-frying or using a microwave are also quick methods that can yield delicious results, if done correctly.

How to Stir-Fry:

Stir-frying is a way to cook small pieces of meat, fish, poultry or vegetables as quickly as possible over very high heat. This seals in the flavor and nutrients while giving the food proper cooking time and minimizing the amount of oil used. Use a heavy iron skillet, electric skillet or wok. I prefer a wok since it's easy to use and clean. The average stir-fry dish takes between three and five minutes of cooking time.

First, prepare all the ingredients and sauce before starting to cook. Cut the food into pieces of similar size to increase the exposed cooking surface. Stir frying is always done with small pieces because the cooking time is so short. Preheat the large skillet or wok over high heat until it just begins to smoke. Use nonstick cooking spray or about 1 to 1.5 tablespoons of olive oil. Pour the oil in a circular motion around the top of the wok or skillet. It will flow to the bottom, coating the sides as it goes. Canola or peanut oil are traditionally used because of the high burning point, but I prefer olive oil. To test the temperature of the oil, add a piece of vegetable; if it sizzles, you are ready to cook.

Cook the seasonings first (garlic, onion, ginger, etc...). They flavor the oil and thus, whatever you add subsequently. Cook the seasonings for about 15 seconds, or until very fragrant, stirring and tossing with a spatula. Add the main ingredients in order of approximate cooking times. It is best to add the meat first, then the hard vegetables such as carrots and cabbage, and then soft vegetables such as squash. Stir-fry these ingredients for one to two minutes or until they are tender-crisp, tossing with a spatula. Keep the food moving to prevent scorching.

The last step is to add the sauce. Bring the mixture to a boil and simmer for a minute or so. Make sure all the ingredients are fully cooked. Taste the stir-fry before serving to correct the seasoning. Add a splash of soy sauce, a squeeze of lemon, or other flavorings to your taste.

Microwave Cooking:

Microwave cooking is a natural part of a healthy lifestyle and makes meal preparation a breeze provided you get it right. Here are six useful tips when using a microwave:

1. When a recipe tells you to cover the food tightly, use either a tight fitting lid recommended for microwaving or plastic wrap. Covering keeps food from drying out.
2. As with stir frying, small pieces cook faster.
3. Don't add salt before microwaving. It can result in food that has a tough, rubbery consistency.
4. Vegetables: For even cooking, make sure they are cut into uniform sizes. A good guide to microwaving fresh vegetables is to allow six minutes per pound.
5. Beef: Different techniques are suited to different cuts of meat. Tender beef should be dry-roasted uncovered on a microwave rack while tougher cuts require liquid and are microwaved tightly covered at a lower power level to help tenderize. Use herbs, spices and citrus juices because not only are you enhancing the flavor of meats, but the acid they contain helps tenderize the meat.
6. Fish: When microwaving, check the fish after the minimum cooking time to see if it's done. Fish will continue to cook after it is removed from the microwave and overcooked fish simply doesn't taste good. Also, if you use the microwave oven to defrost frozen fish,

remember it defrosts quickly. If you overdo it, the fish will toughen.

Fish Ideas

Since fish is such a big part of the Greenwich Diet, I thought I'd share with you some of my marinade ideas. Try any one of the following simple sauces for basting or marinating broiled or steamed seafood.

◆ *Fresh Lemon or Lime Juice*

Squeeze a small amount of fresh lemon or lime juice directly on the fish or seafood.

◆ *Seasoned Lemon Baste*

Combine lemon juice with a dash or two of white wine or vermouth, soy sauce, and/or seasonings of your choice such as dill weed, mustard, pepper, rosemary or thyme.

◆ *Italian-Style Marinade*

Marinate fish for 30 minutes in Italian salad dressing and then broil.

◆ *Honey-Curry Baste or Marinade*

Marinate fish for 15 to 30 minutes, turning occasionally in a marinade containing 1/3 to 1/2 cup soy sauce, 2 tsp. oil, 1 packet of sugar substitute, 2 tsp. lemon juice, 1/2 to 1 tsp. ground ginger, 1/2 to 1 tsp. minced garlic and 2 Tbs. sherry. This makes enough for one to two pounds of fish.

◆ *Garlic-Rosemary Marinade*

Combine ingredients of marinade and pour over one pound of halibut, swordfish or other fish steaks.

Marinate for 35 to 40 minutes and broil or grill. Marinade contains: 2 tsp. olive oil, 1/4 cup fresh lemon juice, 2 cloves minced garlic, 1 Tbs. minced parsley and 1-1/2 Tbs. fresh rosemary sprigs.

Using Herbs & Spices:

The seasonings you add to foods are important. The right ones in the right amounts enhance the flavor of the food. The wrong ones or wrong amounts destroy the flavor. The tips that follow should help you avoid making a mistake.

Check out the following "dos" and "don'ts" of using herbs and seasonings:

DOs	DONTs
◆ Go easy. In general, 1/4 teaspoon of dried herbs or spice is enough for 4 servings.	◆ Don't use the same amounts of fresh and dried herbs. In most cases, 1 teaspoon of dried herb is equal to 3 teaspoons of fresh herbs.
◆ After measuring the correct amount of herbs, crush the herbs in the palm of your hand before adding them to your recipe.	◆ Don't use too many different seasonings in one dish—unless it is a thoroughly tested recipe.
◆ Add dried herbs and seasonings to foods such as salad dressings, fruits and juices, well before you want to serve the food. This allows the flavors plenty of time to blend together.	◆ Don't add dried herbs or seasonings too early. Wait until the last hour of cooking before you add your seasonings.
◆ Balance out seasonings. If your main dish is strongly flavored, use lighter seasoning on your salad and keep your vegetable and desert quite simple.	◆ Don't use herbs or spices in every dish you serve at a meal.

The chart that follows should help you narrow down which spices to use on a particular food. Keep in mind that there are no absolute rules here. It's all about you and what you like. Don't be afraid to experiment. These are just guidelines to get you started, but recommendations I think will work well for you.

Beef	Dry mustard, marjoram, onion, sage, thyme, bay leaf, celery seed, rosemary, green pepper, garlic, mushrooms
Chicken	Basil, chervil, marjoram, tarragon, paprika, thyme, sage, parsley, mushrooms
Lamb	Marjoram, mint, garlic, rosemary, curry
Veal	Rosemary, bay leaf, ginger, marjoram, curry, mushrooms, oregano, paprika
Fish	Basil, chervil, marjoram, tarragon, dry mustard, paprika, curry, green pepper, lemon, dill, mushrooms
Eggs	Basil, marjoram, tarragon, green pepper, mushrooms, dry mustard, paprika, curry
Green beans	Dill, green pepper, watercress, caraway
Cabbage	Green pepper, garlic, onion powder, pimento, oregano, chives, tarragon

GREENWICH DIET

Recipes

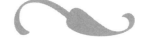

METABOLIFT SUGAR-FREE
HIGH PROTEIN-LOW CARB
FAT-BURNING COFFEE

◆ *16 oz. coffee (Starbucks, 7-Eleven or your preferred brand)*
◆ *One packet Twinlab Metabolift Whey Protein Meal Replacement (preferably chocolate flavor)*
◆ *One packet Equal*
◆ *1 oz. skim milk*

Place approximately one ounce skim milk in empty 16 oz. coffee cup. Stir in one packet of Equal. Add one packet of Metabolift Whey Protein Meal Replacement to skim milk, stirring constantly (about 10 seconds) till mixture reaches the consistency of a paste. Add coffee to cup last, while stirring. Enjoy.

$\mathcal{B}$ROCCOLI ONION CREAM SOUP

- ◆ *1-1/4 pounds finely chopped broccoli*
- ◆ *2-1/2 cans chicken broth*
- ◆ *1 large finely chopped onion*
- ◆ *1/4 tsp. ground black pepper*
- ◆ *1/4 tsp. salt*
- ◆ *1 cup skim milk*

In a large saucepan, over medium-high heat, except for the milk, heat chicken broth, broccoli, onion, salt and pepper to a boil. Reduce heat, cover, and simmer for 30 minutes. Let the mixture cool and in an electric blender under medium speed, add the mixture in batches until a smooth and creamy consistency is achieved. Pour into a large mixing bowl and stir in milk. Chill for an additional hour and serve. This can be served hot or cold. MAKES 5 SERVINGS.

SPINACH-STUFFED TERIYAKI MUSHROOM CAPS

- ◆ *8 oz. fresh spinach*
- ◆ *1-1/2 pounds large mushrooms*
- ◆ *2 tsp. teriyaki sauce*
- ◆ *1/2 cup minced onion*
- ◆ *2 tsp. olive oil*
- ◆ *1-1/2 cups cottage cheese*
- ◆ *2 Tbs. grated Parmesan cheese*
- ◆ *1 tsp. dill*
- ◆ *1/4 tsp. black pepper*
- ◆ *1/4 tsp. salt*

Preheat oven to 400°F. Wash the spinach in cold water and remove any thick stems. Steam spinach, drain, and cool. Next, finely chop all the spinach leaves. Wash mushrooms thoroughly and remove the stems, leaving just the caps. Finely chop the mushroom stems and set them aside. Place the caps round side up on a baking sheet wiped with olive oil. In a large skillet, sauté the onion in the oil until soft. Add chopped mushroom stems and sauté for three minutes. Remove from the heat and stir in the spinach, cottage cheese, Parmesan cheese, dill, teriyaki sauce, salt and pepper. Divide the mixture among the mushroom caps, mounding it. Bake for 20 minutes, or until the tops are lightly browned. MAKES 6 SERVINGS.

*F*RESH SALMON PÂTÉ

- ◆ *8 oz. can fresh boneless salmon*
- ◆ *1-1/2 pounds large mushrooms*
- ◆ *1/2 cup steamed green beans*
- ◆ *1/3 cup cottage cheese*
- ◆ *3 Tbs. diced pimiento*
- ◆ *3 Tbs. chopped onion*
- ◆ *1 Tbs. fresh lemon juice*
- ◆ *1 clove fresh minced garlic*
- ◆ *1/4 tsp. Tabasco*

Place salmon in a blender with all other ingredients. Blend well. Pour into a mold and chill for at least four hours. Serve with vegetables. MAKES 2 CUPS.

SPINACH FETA OMELET

- ◆ *5 oz. fresh shredded spinach leaves*
- ◆ *1/4 cup water*
- ◆ *2 Tbs. feta cheese*
- ◆ *4 eggs*
- ◆ *1-1/2 tsp. olive oil*

In a large covered saucepan, over medium heat, cook spinach and water for three minutes or until spinach is wilted. Drain thoroughly and add crumbled cheese. Set this aside and add whisked eggs to large frying pan lined with olive oil (hint: never add oil to a cold pan). Cook over medium heat, lifting edges to allow the uncooked portion to flow underneath. When almost set, spoon spinach mixture over half the omelet. Fold other half over filling. If you're feeling brave, try flipping it. Otherwise, wait a couple of seconds and simply slide it onto a dish and serve immediately. (Trying to eat a cold omelet is a brutal experience). MAKES 2 SERVINGS.

TANGY FLAX SALAD DRESSING

- ◆ *1/2 cup red wine vinegar*
- ◆ *1/4 cup liquid flaxseed oil*
- ◆ *1/4 cup balsamic vinegar*
- ◆ *1/4 tsp. ground pepper*
- ◆ *1/2 tsp. salt*
- ◆ *1 packet, sugar substitute*
- ◆ *2 cloves garlic (crushed)*
- ◆ *2 tsp. Worcestershire sauce*

Mix the ingredients together in an appropriately sized cruet and shake well. Then add 1/2 cup water and shake again. MAKES ABOUT 1-1/2 CUPS.

*S*wiss asparagus frittata

- ◆ *6 eggs*
- ◆ *1/2 cup shredded Swiss cheese*
- ◆ *1/4 cup skim milk*
- ◆ *1 Tbs. olive oil*
- ◆ *6 spears fresh asparagus*
- ◆ *1 large onion*
- ◆ *1 tsp. fresh rosemary leaves*
- ◆ *1/4 tsp. ground black pepper*

Preheat oven broiler. Combine eggs, cheese and milk, whisk thoroughly, and set aside. In a 10-inch ovenproof skillet, over medium-high heat, cook and stir finely diced asparagus, chopped onion, rosemary, and pepper in olive oil for three minutes. Make sure to add the onions first. Reduce heat to low, then pour egg mixture evenly into the skillet over the vegetable mixture. Cover and cook for 12 minutes. Remove cover and place under a preheated broiler for three minutes or until set. Cut into wedges and serve. MAKES 6 SERVINGS.

KALE SEA SALAD

- ◆ *2 cups kale (torn)*
- ◆ *1 pound asparagus spears (chopped)*
- ◆ *1/4 cup shallots (diced)*
- ◆ *1 cup water*
- ◆ *1 Tbs. olive oil*
- ◆ *1 Tbs. balsamic vinegar*
- ◆ *12 fresh clams (scrubbed and in their shells)*
- ◆ *12 fresh mussels (scrubbed and in their shells)*
- ◆ *1/2 cup sweet red and yellow peppers (minced)*
- ◆ *2 Tbs. parsley (minced)*

In a large pot of boiling water, blanch the asparagus for two minutes, then drain and set aside. In a 4-quart pot, sauté the shallots in the olive oil for four minutes. Add the water and vinegar and heat to boiling. Add the clams, then cover and cool for 1-1/2 minutes. Add the mussels; cover and cook for five minutes until all the shells open. Remove and discard the shells (discard any unopened shells). Place the clams and mussels in a large bowl. Sprinkle with parsley. Pour the cooking liquid over the shellfish, being careful not to transfer any sediment or sand that ends up on the bottom of the pot. (Having sand in your salad is worse than having a shell in your eggs!) Divide the asparagus, kale and peppers among individual dinner plates and spoon on the shellfish mixture. Serve warm or at room temperature. MAKES 4 SERVINGS.

$\mathcal{M}$ONACO SALAD

- ◆ *2 cups romaine lettuce (chopped)*
- ◆ *2 cups bok choy (chopped)*
- ◆ *1/2 cup endive (chopped)*
- ◆ *1/2 cup spinach (remove stems and chop)*
- ◆ *1/2 cup red cabbage (chopped)*
- ◆ *1/2 cup cucumbers (peeled and sliced)*
- ◆ *1/2 cup celery (sliced)*
- ◆ *1/2 cup mushrooms (sliced)*
- ◆ *1/4 cup carrot shreds*

Mix all the vegetables together and toss. This salad is best served with a poppy seed dressing. MAKES 4 SERVINGS.

SHRIMP AND SPINACH MUSTARD SALAD

◆ *1 pound medium-sized fresh shrimp (peeled, de-veined and steamed)*
◆ *1/2 cup Dijon mustard*
◆ *1 packet sugar substitute*
◆ *1 tsp. brown sugar*
◆ *1 Tbs. balsamic vinegar*
◆ *3 cups romaine lettuce (shredded)*
◆ *3 cups spinach (shredded)*
◆ *1 small red onion (sliced)*
◆ *1 large cucumber (sliced)*
◆ *1/3 cup shelled pecans (broken up into pieces)*

For dressing, combine mustard, honey, brown sugar, lime juice and vinegar; chill until serving time. On a large serving platter, layer lettuce leaves, spinach, onion slices, cucumber slices, and shrimp. To serve, sprinkle with pecans and drizzle with prepared salad dressing. MAKES 6 SERVINGS.

SHRIMP GARLIC SAUTE

- ◆ *30 jumbo shrimp*
- ◆ *2 Tbs. virgin olive oil*
- ◆ *4 cloves garlic (minced)*
- ◆ *2 large onions (chopped)*
- ◆ *5 sweet red peppers (cut into thin strips)*
- ◆ *2 tomatoes (cored and chopped)*
- ◆ *1/4 tsp. salt*
- ◆ *1/4 tsp. pepper*

Sauté shrimp in 1 Tbs. olive oil and 1 clove garlic until cooked, then set it aside. In a large, deep skillet that has a cover, heat 1 Tbs. olive oil, then add the garlic and onions. Sauté for one minute and add the sweet pepper strips. Cook for one minute and stir. Cover the pan and simmer over low heat for about 10 minutes. Remove cover and add the tomatoes. Continue cooking the mixture over moderately low heat for another five minutes. Stir occasionally. Add salt and pepper. Serve hot, chilled, or at room temperature. SERVES 6.

OLIVE STUFFED FLOUNDER

- ◆ 2 cups broccoli (chopped)
- ◆ 1/3 cup onion (chopped)
- ◆ 1 clove garlic (minced)
- ◆ 12 medium green olives (with pimento)
- ◆ 1 Tbs. olive oil
- ◆ 1/3 cup plain whole-wheat bread crumbs
- ◆ 1/4 cup red pepper (chopped)
- ◆ 1 egg
- ◆ 6 4-oz. flounder fillets
- ◆ 2 Tbs. lime juice
- ◆ chopped parsley and lemon slices for garnish

Preheat oven to 375°F. In a skillet, over medium heat, cook broccoli, onion and garlic in oil until tender. Remove from heat; cool slightly. Stir in bread crumbs, red pepper, olives and egg. Spoon stuffing onto one end of fillet; roll up fillet, encasing stuffing. Arrange in 11x7x1.5-inch baking dish; sprinkle with lime juice. Bake for 15 to 20 minutes until fish flakes easily when tested with a fork. Garnish with parsley and lemon slices. MAKES 6 SERVINGS.

PENNSYLVANIA PEPPERCORN POT ROAST

- ◆ *Cooking spray*
- ◆ *1-1/2 pounds beef (eye round preferred)*
- ◆ *1 cup beef broth*
- ◆ *1 cup chopped onion*
- ◆ *1/2 cup canned crushed tomatoes with added puree (undrained)*
- ◆ *1/4 cup diced carrots*
- ◆ *1/4 cup diced celery*
- ◆ *1/4 cup diced turnip*
- ◆ *2 Tbs. fresh parsley (chopped)*
- ◆ *1/4 tsp. dried thyme*
- ◆ *6 black peppercorns*

Place a large saucepan, coated with cooking spray, over medium-high heat until hot. Add roast, browning on all sides. Add broth, onions, tomatoes, carrots, celery, turnip, parsley and thyme. Bring to a boil. Add peppercorns. Cover, reduce heat, and simmer three hours or until tender. Remove roast from saucepan and slice; place on a serving platter. Set aside; keep warm. Reheat saucepan; increase heat to medium. Cook broth mixture, uncovered, 10 minutes or until reduced to about 1-2/3 cups. Discard peppercorns. Serve sauce with roast. MAKES 5 SERVINGS.

NEW ORLEANS CAJUN CATFISH

- ♦ *1/4 cup buttermilk*
- ♦ *3 tsp. Dijon mustard*
- ♦ *3/4 cup crumbled whole-wheat crackers*
- ♦ *1 tsp. salt*
- ♦ *1-1/2 tsp. paprika*
- ♦ *1 tsp. onion powder*
- ♦ *1 tsp. garlic powder*
- ♦ *1/2 tsp. dried thyme leaves*
- ♦ *1 tsp. ground red pepper*
- ♦ *4 catfish fillets (medium)*
- ♦ *1 large lemon*

Preheat the broiler. Oil a wire rack large enough to hold the fish in a single layer. Put the rack on a baking sheet and set aside. In a medium bowl, whisk the buttermilk and mustard together until it forms a smooth consistency. In a shallow bowl, combine the cracker crumbles, salt, paprika, onion powder, garlic powder, thyme, and pepper. Dip each fillet in the buttermilk mixture, turning to coat. Transfer to the crumbled cracker mixture, turning to coat completely. Place the fillets on the prepared rack. Broil approximately four inches from the heat source until the fish is opaque in the center (about three minutes per side). Serve hot with lemon wedges. SERVES 4.

Southwestern spicy chicken sauté

- ◆ *1 Tbs. chili powder*
- ◆ *1-1/2 tsp. cumin*
- ◆ *1/4 tsp. salt*
- ◆ *1/4 tsp. ground red pepper*
- ◆ *4 chicken breasts (boneless)*
- ◆ *2 tsp. olive oil*
- ◆ *1/2 cup chicken broth (defatted)*
- ◆ *1 Tbs. cider vinegar*
- ◆ *1 large yellow onion (chopped)*
- ◆ *1 4-oz. can green chilies (rinsed and drained)*
- ◆ *1/4 cup fresh cilantro (chopped)*
- ◆ *1 lime (cut into wedges)*

In a cup, mix the chili powder, cumin, salt and red pepper. Rub both sides of the chicken breasts with 1 tablespoon of the spice mixture. In a large, heavy, non-stick skillet, warm the oil over medium-high heat. Add the chicken and sauté for two to three minutes on each side, or until the spice coating is browned and the surface of the chicken is opaque. Remove chicken and set aside. Add the onions to the skillet and lightly brown them. Add broth, vinegar and remaining spice mixture to the skillet. Increase the heat to high and bring to a boil, stirring occasionally. Boil for two minutes. Return the chicken to the skillet. Add the chilies and bring to a simmer. Spoon the chili mixture over the chicken; reduce the heat to medium. Cover and simmer for six minutes, making sure the chicken is cooked through. Transfer to a serving dish and garnish with the fresh cilantro and lime wedges. MAKES 4 SERVINGS.

*H*ARVEST BAKED ACORN SQUASH

- ◆ *2 medium acorn squash (about 1-1/2 pounds each)*
- ◆ *2 cups apple (finely chopped)*
- ◆ *1/4 cup apple juice*
- ◆ *1 Tbs. olive oil*
- ◆ *1 packet of sugar substitute*
- ◆ *2 tsp. lemon juice*
- ◆ *3/4 tsp. ground cinnamon*
- ◆ *3/4 cup coarsely crushed whole grain or oat crackers*
- ◆ *1 tsp. ground nutmeg*

Preheat oven to 400°F. Cut squash in half crosswise and remove seeds. Place in a 13x9x2-inch baking dish and fill with water to 1/2-inch depth. Bake for 45 minutes. Scoop the cooked squash out of shells and place contents into a bowl. Put shells aside. Combine squash, apples, apple juice, olive oil, honey, lemon juice, and cinnamon. Try to do this while the squash is still warm. Again, while still warm, stir in crushed crackers. Spoon squash mixture into shells; sprinkle with nutmeg. Bake for 10 minutes more, or until hot. MAKES 4 SERVINGS.

Pepper Rockfish

- ◆ *1 cup mixed herbs (parsley, sage, basil, chives), coarsely chopped*
- ◆ *1/4 tsp. salt*
- ◆ *1/2 tsp. freshly ground black pepper*
- ◆ *4 4-oz. rockfish filets (skinless)*
- ◆ *1 egg white*

Sprinkle the herbs, salt and pepper on a large platter. Brush each rockfish fillet with the egg white (whisked first), then dredge in the herbs. In a large nonstick skillet over medium-high heat, sear the fillets three to four minutes on each side until cooked through. SERVES 4.

CANTONESE FLOUNDER

- ◆ *4 scallions (cut into thin 2" strips)*
- ◆ *2-inch piece of ginger root (peeled and cut into thin 2" strips)*
- ◆ *4 4-oz. flounder fillets*
- ◆ *2 Tbs. low sodium soy sauce*
- ◆ *2 Tbs. dry sherry*
- ◆ *1 tsp. sesame oil*
- ◆ *1/2 packet sugar substitute*
- ◆ *1/4 tsp. hot chili oil*

Preheat the oven to 375°F. Sprinkle half the scallions and half the ginger into a 9x13-inch baking dish. Place the fillets in the dish, with the side that has the silvery skin facing down. Sprinkle on the remaining scallions and ginger. In a small bowl, combine the soy sauce, sherry, sesame oil, sugar substitute and chili oil and pour the mixture over the fish. Marinate for 15 minutes prior to cooking. Cover the baking dish with foil and place it in the oven. Bake for 15 minutes, until the fish is opaque. SERVES 4.

Coriander chicken

- ◆ *2 cloves garlic (minced)*
- ◆ *1 medium onion (chopped)*
- ◆ *1 Tbs. extra virgin olive oil*
- ◆ *2 chicken breasts (boneless, skinned, halved and cubed)*
- ◆ *2 tsp. ground coriander*
- ◆ *1 tsp. ground ginger*
- ◆ *1/8 tsp. cayenne pepper*
- ◆ *2 cups plain yogurt*
- ◆ *1/4 cup water*
- ◆ *2 Tbs. cornstarch*
- ◆ *1/4 tsp. salt*
- ◆ *1/4 tsp. pepper*

In a large skillet, saute the garlic and onion in the oil until dark golden. Add the chicken and sauté until well browned. Add 1/4 cup water and the coriander, ginger, cumin, cardamom and cayenne. Simmer uncovered for 20 minutes. Stir occasionally until the chicken is cooked (the liquid will be mostly absorbed at this point). Stir the cornstarch into the yogurt gradually until it dissolves, then stir the mixture into the skillet. Simmer, stirring constantly, until the sauce thickens. Do not boil. Season with salt and pepper. SERVES 4.

TANGY SALSA RED SNAPPER

- ◆ *1 pound red snapper fillets*
- ◆ *4 scallions (minced)*
- ◆ *1 green pepper (diced)*
- ◆ *1 sweet yellow pepper (diced)*
- ◆ *1 cup pineapple (diced)*
- ◆ *1/4 cup red onion (diced)*
- ◆ *3 Tbs. lime juice*
- ◆ *1/4 cup water*
- ◆ *1 jalapeño pepper (minced)*
- ◆ *1 clove garlic (minced)*
- ◆ *1 Tbs. extra virgin olive oil*
- ◆ *1/2 tsp. ground coriander*
- ◆ *1/4 tsp. ground black pepper*
- ◆ *1/8 tsp. thyme*
- ◆ *1 tsp. orange rind (grated)*

To make the salsa: Combine all the ingredients in a bowl, except for the snapper; mix thoroughly. Cover and let marinate for one hour in the refrigerator. To make the snapper: Place the fish in a baking dish. Pour the salsa marinade over the fish. Cover and refrigerate for two additional hours. Remove the fish from the salsa marinade and place into a broiler, skin side down. Broil or grill the fish about four inches from the heat for about five minutes. Save the fish marinade in a separate container. Carefully flip the fish and brush with the marinade and cook for another five minutes or until cooked through. Serve with the salsa marinade. SERVES 4.

SHERRY MUSHROOM CHICKEN

- ◆ *2 large whole boneless chicken breasts*
- ◆ *1 cup chicken broth*
- ◆ *20 whole-wheat crackers (crushed into crumbs)*
- ◆ *1 tsp. basil leaves (dried)*
- ◆ *1 egg*
- ◆ *2 Tbs. olive oil*
- ◆ *1/2 cup dry sherry*
- ◆ *2 Tbs. parsley (chopped)*
- ◆ *1 Tbs. lime juice*
- ◆ *2 cups mushrooms (sliced)*
- ◆ *1/2 tsp. garlic powder*

In a pie plate, combine crumbs, basil and garlic powder. Pound chicken breasts to 1/4-inch thickness. Dip chicken in egg, then coat with crumb mixture. In a 10-inch skillet, over medium heat, brown chicken in 1 Tbs. olive oil until cooked and golden on each side, about 10 minutes. Remove from skillet to serving platter; keep warm. Blend chicken broth, sherry, parsley and lime juice. Add mushrooms and broth mixture to skillet. Heat until mixture thickens and begins to boil and mushrooms are tender; serve over chicken. MAKES 4 SERVINGS.

*L*EMON OREGANO CHICKEN

- *1/2 cup fresh-squeezed lemon juice*
- *3 cloves garlic (finely chopped)*
- *1 Tbs. fresh oregano (chopped) or 1 tsp. dried*
- *1/2 Tbs. ground cinnamon*
- *1/2 tsp. tomato paste or ketchup*
- *4 chicken breasts trimmed of fat*
- *4 sprigs fresh oregano*

In a large dish, combine the lemon juice, garlic, chopped oregano, cinnamon and tomato paste or ketchup. Add chicken and coat well. Cover with plastic wrap and marinate in the refrigerator for at least two hours (six hours maximum), turning occasionally. Prepare a grill or preheat the broiler. Drain the marinade from the chicken. Grill or broil the chicken on a lightly oiled rack until cooked (about six minutes per side). Garnish with the fresh sprigs of oregano. SERVES 4.

"BEARLY" SALMON

- ◆ 2 Tbs. low sodium soy sauce
- ◆ 2 cloves garlic (minced)
- ◆ 1 Tbs. lemon juice
- ◆ 1 packet sugar substitute
- ◆ 4 4-oz. salmon fillets
- ◆ 1/2 cup sun-dried tomatoes (chopped)
- ◆ 1/2 cup water
- ◆ 1/2 tsp. ground cumin
- ◆ 1/4 cup green onions (chopped)
- ◆ 1/4 cup fresh cilantro (chopped)

To make the marinade: In a shallow glass baking dish, combine the soy sauce, garlic, lemon juice and sugar substitute. Add the salmon filets, cover, refrigerate, and marinate for three hours. To make the sauce: In a saucepan over medium-high heat combine the tomatoes, water, and cumin. Bring to a boil, reduce the heat to low, and simmer until the tomatoes are soft (about 10 minutes). Add the green onions and cilantro and mix well. Next, remove the salmon from the marinade and discard the remaining marinade. In a large frying pan over medium-high heat, add the salmon to the pan and sauté for approximately three minutes on one side. Turn and sauté the fish on the other side for another three minutes just until it separates with a fork. Top each fillet with sauce and serve. SERVES 4.

PEPPER TUNA SASHIMI

- ◆ *10 ounces raw 2-inch thick block tuna (must be perfectly fresh)*
- ◆ *2 Tbs. coarse black pepper*
- ◆ *1 Tbs. ground white pepper*
- ◆ *2 Tbs. olive oil*
- ◆ *2 Tbs. fresh ginger (grated)*
- ◆ *1/4 cup low sodium soy sauce*

Mix peppers in a small bowl and spill out onto a clean surface. Coat the block tuna in the pepper, gently pressing the block into the mix. When well coated, you're ready to cook. Heat a medium-sized frying pan to medium-high heat. Add two tablespoons of olive oil to the pan. With a set of prongs, pick up the tuna and place it in the center of the pan on one side of the block. Keep the tuna in place until that particular end is well seared (about 20 seconds). Do the same to each side until the entire exterior of the tuna block is well seared. Remove the tuna and let it cool momentarily on a cutting block. Proceed with a very sharp knife to cut the tuna into thin slices. The outside should be well cooked, while the inside should be raw. Serve with soy sauce and ginger on the side. This dish is an excellent appetizer, but also works well as a main course when served with fresh green beans lightly sautéed in olive oil, lemon and salt. SERVES 2.

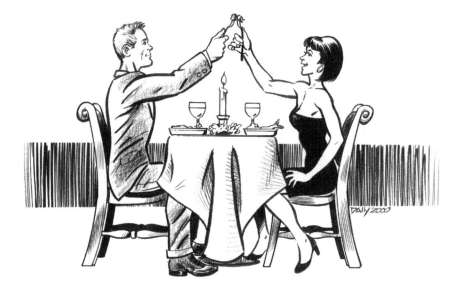

Dining Out On the Greenwich Diet

Staying consistent with the Greenwich Diet while dining out is remarkably easy. This comes as a surprise to those who have tried other diets and have been unable to find things to eat at a restaurant. When dining out "Greenwich-style," keep an eye out for food choices that fit the principles you've learned and look for these items on the restaurant menu. The following table will help start you off in terms of what to look for when heading out to eat, while the breakdown of types of dining by ethnicity that follows should make the whole concept of dining out "easy as pie." (Sorry, I just couldn't resist the pun!)

Appetizers
Vegetables, shrimp or other seafood cocktail, oysters, steamed clams or mussels.

Soups
Vegetable, consommé, broth, plain onion, other broth-based soups.

Salads
Tossed green salad, spinach salad, cottage cheese, chicken, seafood, or egg salad.

Salad Dressings
Olive oil and balsamic vinegar, regular or sugar-free salad dressing, lemon juice.

Meat
Filet mignon, beef round, sirloin or tenderloin.

Poultry
Chicken or turkey breast (broiled or baked). Specify that no butter or lard be used in cooking.

Fish
Any variety (poached, baked or broiled). Olive oil may be used in the cooking.

Desserts
Sugar-free Jell-O, low-fat cheeses.

Beverages
Water, Diet Snapple® iced tea, sugar-free flavored seltzer water, Diet Coke® soda. Coffee and tea in moderation.

Avoid the following:
Potatoes, rice, pasta, bread, sugar-containing desserts, and fruit plates.

American

American restaurants are all the types of places offering traditional American favorites with no particular ethnic emphasis. The range is quite broad, but includes everything from highway diners to fancy colonial inns. Either way, finding something to eat is easy.

Appetizers:

• Tossed side salad
• Chicken broth

Entrées:
- Grilled chicken breast with vegetables
- Swordfish broiled with lemon and olive oil with vegetables
- Lobster with lemon and vegetables with olive oil
- Filet mignon, shell steak, well-trimmed prime rib, or strip steak with vegetables
- Dinner salad

Chinese

Choose dishes that are steamed or lightly stir-fried in vegetable oil, rather than deep fried. Ask for dishes that are not deep-fat fried.

Appetizers:
- Egg Drop Soup

Entrées:
- Steamed seafood or chicken with mixed vegetables

French

Sauces:
- Madeira (wine with mushrooms), diable (mustard), bourguignonne (wine).

Entrées:
- Tournedos (filet of beef)
- Rack of lamb (chops)
- Scallops of veal
- Coq au vin (chicken with red wine)
- Poulet au fines herbs (roast chicken with herbs)
- Lobster, baked or broiled

Greek/Middle Eastern

Most of these dishes are prepared with olive oil. Don't overdo the lamb in Middle Eastern restaurants because it is usually quite fatty. Many of the dishes rely greatly on meat, with appetizers offering vegetable selections.

Entrées:
- Greek salad
- Tzatzeki (cucumber and yogurt sauce)
- Shish kebab (beef, lamb, or chicken with onions and peppers)
- Gyros (lamb and beef served with lettuce, onions, and tzateki sauce). *Hint: Get it without the pita bread.*
- Dolma (grape leaves stuffed with ground lamb, onions and spices). This is okay as long as you stay away from the ones with all the rice.

Indian

Many of the dishes use a yogurt-based curry sauce.

Entrées:
- Raita (combination of yogurt with chopped or shredded vegetables)
- Tandoori chicken and fish dishes (Be aware that butter is used to baste some of these preparations).
- Shish kebab (marinated ground lamb cooked over coals)
- Vegetable curries and dal

Italian

Sauces:
- Olive oil and garlic

Entrées:
- Chicken
- Veal with mushrooms or veal with lemon or wine
- Beef filet
- Fish/seafood
- Roasted Italian peppers
- All fish, baked, steamed, poached, broiled or bouillabaisse

Japanese

Japanese dishes tend to be lower in fat. Avoid the deep-fried tempura dishes. Look for the word "yakimono," which means broiled.

Appetizers:
- Salad with ginger dressing
- Seaweed salad

Entrées:
- Chicken or fish teriyaki
- Yakitori (chicken)
- Sashimi (raw fish)
- Yakimono (broiled fish and chicken)

Mexican

Avoid the flour and corn tortillas. Having guacamole, salsa or grated cheese on top of your dish is a great way of spicing things up.

Entrées:
- Seviche (fish marinated in lime juice)
- Shrimp or chicken tostados without the tortilla or rice

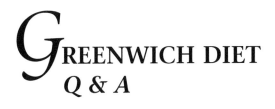

GREENWICH DIET
Q & A

The following questions and answers represent the most commonly discussed concerns from our clients at our clinic in Greenwich, Connecticut.

Q. *Is the Greenwich Diet a "diet" or more of a healthy eating plan?*

A. The Greenwich Diet is more of a healthy eating plan versus a "diet." It consists of various foods and offers one options for meals and snacks. In so doing, rather than restricting intake, we look to educate the client in terms of what foods will be healthier choices. As a result, no true Greenwich Dieter ever really feels like they are dieting.

Q. *When I think of the word "diet" I think of a grapefruit for breakfast and a shake for lunch and dinner; in other words, little amounts of food with no variety. Is that going to be the case?*

A. No, quite the contrary. Many of the clients that have

been on the Greenwich diet are baffled by the fact that they are often required to eat more meals than they are used to, yet they lose weight! Although fat seems to melt off your body, you are absolutely not starving yourself. There is a plethora of easily accessible foods that are what we call "Greenwich Diet compliant," and offer tremendous variety, flavor and eating enjoyment.

Q. *How long does it take to lose weight and see results on the Greenwich Diet?*

A. Beyond the first few days of adjustment, within only one week of following the Greenwich Diet, you will most probably see a significant loss in weight while feeling more energized. Within a couple of months of following the Greenwich Diet, your big complaint will be that your tailoring bill is so high, or that you had to spend money on a new wardrobe! Sorry, but it's a small price to pay for a healthy, beautiful body.

Q. *Does everyone lose weight on the Greenwich Diet?*

A. Because over half the population in America is overweight or obese according to a recent study published in the *Journal of the American Medical Association*, you are nearly guaranteed to lose weight. The weight that is lost is fat, not lean muscle.

Q. *By following the Greenwich Diet, how easily will I lose the fat on my body?*

A. As long as you follow the guidelines and rules of the Greenwich Diet, you should find that your body easily drops off the fat. The degree to which you burn fat depends on how much fat you have on your body and the severity of your weight problem. Heavier people lose considerably more fat than thinner people simply because they have more to lose.

Q. *Should my physician know that I'm on the Greenwich Diet?*

A. We believe knowledge is power. Always letting your physician know what you are doing with your body is wise and responsible. Prudence in healthcare is paramount. But don't be surprised if your physician doesn't know much about the diet. I hate to admit it, but many of my colleagues are behind the times on this subject. Just be gentle. Giving your physician a copy of the book is a good way to familiarize him or her with the sensibility of what you are doing, while giving others the opportunity to share in the benefits of the Greenwich Diet.

Q. *Do I have to take supplements on the Greenwich Diet?*

A. You do not have to take supplements on the Greenwich Diet. However, I strongly encourage you to at least take the basic supplements referred to in the book. In particular, the Metabolift Whey Protein Meal Replacement, Metabolift multivitamin and TwinEPA (fish oil) are of quintessential importance. Other supplements really depend on your individual needs, goals and desires. Supplementing the diet makes dieting easier to comply with and healthier in terms of insuring that vital nutrients are not missed.

Q. *If I splurge on a big pasta dinner with garlic bread, will I gain all the weight back that I've lost?*

A. Don't worry so much! Splurging occasionally on carbohydrate-rich foods won't ruin your life and certainly will not put back all the weight you've lost. However, depending on how long you have been on the diet, you may feel bloated and fatigued after a high carbohydrate meal since you won't be used to eating that way. All the better! It will make you crave carbohydrates even less. As long as heavy carbohydrate sessions are kept to a minimum and you get back on track the next day, things won't change for the worse.

Q. *Can I ever eat pasta, bread, rice and other carbohydrates again on a regular basis?*

A. Simply stated, no. When you initially begin the Greenwich Diet you want to avoid them until you start losing weight. Once you get to the maintenance stage of the Greenwich Diet, you can incorporate them on rare occasion, but more than likely and as already mentioned, you won't crave them. Having carbohydrate-based meals is a big problem, so I want you to break out of the habit and make healthier food choices. Carbohydrates are a narcotic to which America is addicted. The Greenwich Diet detoxifies the body from sugar overload and finally relieves the body of these unhealthy and unnatural cravings.

Q. *I usually don't have breakfast in the morning. Do I have to eat breakfast on the Greenwich Diet?*

A. One of the first things we teach you on the Greenwich Diet is the importance of the morning meal. Most people on poor diets are conditioned not to eat in the morning, and thus have no appetite when they wake up. Greenwich Dieters learn to eat first thing in the morning because it is a natural feeding time. Your body is desperately in need of nutrients after an overnight fast. Avoiding breakfast, is like a car running on vapors! The same holds true for your body. Without an early first meal, your metabolism can't run efficiently for very long and you will quickly slip into the condition of starvation alert. This meal is your body's first source of replenishment. It sets the body at ease and paves a way for a positive interaction with food the rest of the day.

Q. *Once I start, do I have to stay on the Greenwich Diet the rest of my life?*

A. I hate to use the word "diet" when referring to the Greenwich Diet, but it seems to have become the industry standard when describing specific ways of eating. Keep in mind that the Greenwich Diet is a healthy eating plan that teaches you about making better food choices. Once past detoxifying your body from the narcotic influence of carbohydrates, adding whey protein, replenishing water, increasing dietary fiber and adding essential nutrient fat, the Greenwich Diet won't seem like a diet at all. Your body will be refreshed and energized. You will be eating plenty of food and almost never be hungry. The cravings for junk food and sugar will subside and you will be on a course toward gaining new health and wellness. You might find yourself occasionally eating foods that are not on the Greenwich Diet, but that's okay. The struggle will be over. You will be able to effortlessly control yourself because the cravings simply won't be there. For example, if you were to make several conscious choices of foods not on the Greenwich Diet, you would do them knowingly. You would then simply compensate for them by following-up this noncompliance with a series of better food choices. As a result, you would be back on track with ease and control.

Q. *How long should I stay on the Greenwich Diet?*

A. Although the Greenwich Diet seems to literally melt the fat off your body in effortless fashion and in record time, I still view it as being more of a healthy eating plan than a fat burning diet. Remember, learn and be educated. Let the diet "speak" to you. In a short time you will learn more about your body and make small adjustments within the diet to insure easy long-term compliance. The Greenwich Diet is an education for life.

S UPPORTING SCIENCE *and* CASE REPORTS

XI

Our clinical team of physician, registered dietitians, and physiologists has extensively researched the Greenwich Diet. We have carefully monitored large numbers of clients throughout years of the program at my clinic, Peak Wellness, Inc., in Greenwich, Connecticut. We've seen extraordinary weight loss, body fat loss and muscle maintenance in those individuals on the diet. In addition, increased energy levels and healthier cholesterol and triglyceride levels were noted in participants.

In fact, 43 people with a BMI (body mass index) greater than 25 were followed on the Greenwich Diet over a period of six months. All of them, without exception, experienced a significant improvement in body weight, body fat, cholesterol, triglycerides and/or energy levels. Currently, the Greenwich Diet is being researched in comparison to the *American Heart Association* Step I Diet. Fifty people are being examined, 25 in each group. Body composition changes, coronary risk profile, blood sugar, profile of mood states, among a host of other parameters, are being examined. Early results already show a great advantage in those on the Greenwich Diet. The results will be published next year in a peer-reviewed scientific journal.

The case reports that follow represent typical real-life examples of people from our clinic. They are not simply isolated success stories of extreme cases. Rather, they are typical stories of real people like you that we see every day as patients and clients of our clinic.

CASE REPORT 1

RS, a 68-year-old male college professor with 30 pounds to lose, came to us a victim of recurrent dietary failure using virtually all the popular methods. He was being medicated for high blood pressure and gout. Additionally, he was repeatedly ill with minor but equally annoying upper respiratory infections and sore throats. These infections would frequently keep him out of work. As a result, he was drawing sharp criticism from his colleagues who claimed that as a result of his "advancing years," he was perpetually ill and unfit to meet the demands of educating college students. After only five weeks on the Greenwich Diet he lost 25 pounds. After two months, he no longer needed medications of any kind. In fact, his blood pressure had normalized without any pills. Interestingly, by the third month, he was no longer experiencing weekly upper respiratory infections and sore throats. I understand he hasn't missed a day's work since and, as a result, muzzled his critics.

CASE REPORT 2

BG was only 29 years old when she first came in, but she suffered from morbid obesity and the beginnings of early diabetes. She was a very pretty lady with model-like features, but at only 5'4" she weighed close to 200 pounds. After only five weeks of the Greenwich Diet she had lost nearly 35 pounds. Quickly gaining confidence from this early success, and seeing her blood sugar completely normalize, she stayed very compliant and went on to lose an additional 30 pounds in the subsequent two months. So far, she has managed to keep it off effortlessly and it's been almost a year. I also hear she's doing some modeling.

CASE REPORT 3

BH, a 42-year-old wealthy male investment banker, came in complaining of having "excess baggage" around his waist. Although not terribly obese, he did have about 15 pounds to lose. He complained that with all the traveling he does combined with mandatory evening dinner meetings for business, dieting was impossible. Upon careful questioning, it was also revealed that he was chronically constipated, with only a single bowel movement in as many as three days. Shortly after starting the Greenwich Diet, he was able to adjust his eating properly and make better choices. Interestingly, but not surprisingly, if you understand the concepts of the diet, he ended up eating more total calories throughout the day, yet dropped 12 pounds in less than three weeks. He also began experiencing regular daily bowel movements—a small but important relief that BH will be the first to admit money can't buy.

CASE REPORT 4

RF is a 34-year-old small business owner who was 40 pounds overweight when he started the Greenwich Diet. His biggest complaint, apart from the excess weight, was an apparent need for sleeping nearly twelve hours a night, extreme difficulty waking-up, and sluggishness throughout the day. He felt quite strongly that the poor performance of his business was directly related to his lack of productive working hours. After seven weeks on the Greenwich Diet he had dropped the entire 40 pounds. Waking up with ease at nearly 5 a.m. every morning and seldom requiring more than six hours of sleep each night, he was finally able to work substantive, energetic days. As a result, the size of his business literally doubled, while his waistline practically halved!

CASE REPORT 5

At 45 years of age, despite a lifetime of great physical activity including two completed marathons, as well as being an avid tennis player, swimmer and golfer, KN couldn't seem to get rid of the cellulite on her legs and buttocks. She blamed it on her genetics and felt resigned to her fate since a life of being athletic didn't seem to make much of a difference. Then she discovered the Greenwich Diet. As a result of her dietary compliance, she was able to identify and break away from her dependence on carbohydrates as an energy source. Finally, she was able to get control of her body and tone her previously unresponsive physique. The results remain unbelievable. All of her friends want to know how she did it, her husband is amazed, and she even managed to get compliments from her teenage kids—something she assured me is next to impossible!

CARBOHYDRATE GRAM COUNTER

XII

Foods	Amount	Grams of Carbohydrate
Beverages		
Beer		
Light	8 fl. oz.	3.0
Regular	8 fl. oz.	7.0
Club soda	8 fl. oz.	0
Coffee (black)	8 fl. oz.	0
Grape juice	8 fl. oz.	36.0
Grapefruit juice	8 fl. oz.	23.0
Lemonade, from concentrate	8 fl. oz.	27.0
Milk		
Low-fat (1%)	8 fl. oz.	12.0
Low-fat (2%)	8 fl. oz.	12.0
Skim	8 fl. oz.	12.0
Whole	8 fl. oz.	11.0
Orange juice	8 fl. oz.	26.0
Pineapple juice, unsweetened	8 fl. oz.	34.0
Soda		
Diet	8 fl. oz.	1.0
Regular	8 fl. oz.	26.0
Tea		
Brewed	8 fl. oz.	0
Instant, diet	8 fl. oz.	1.0
Instant, sweetened	8 fl. oz.	22.0
Tomato juice	8 fl. oz.	10.0
Wine		
Champagne	3 fl. oz.	0
Port	3 fl. oz.	11.0
Red wine	3 fl. oz.	3.0
Sherry	3 fl. oz.	11.0
White wine	3 fl. oz.	3.0

Foods	Amount	Grams of Carbohydrate
Breads, bread products, and crackers		
Bagel	1 plain	38.0
Biscuit	1 plain	13.0
Bread crumbs, commercial	1 cup	73.0
Breads		
French, thick slice	1 slice	20.0
Italian	1 slice	17.0
Mixed grain	1 slice	12.0
Pita	1 pita	33.0
Pumpernickel	1 slice	17.0
Raisin	1 slice	13.0
Rye	1 slice	12.0
Wheat	1 slice	12.0
White	1 slice	12.0
Whole wheat	1 slice	13.0
Crackers		
Cheese, sandwich	1 sandwich	5.0
Graham	1 cracker	6.0
Saltines	1 cracker	2.0
Whole wheat	1 cracker	2.0
Croutons, plain	1 oz.	20.0
English muffin, plain	1	27.0
Matzo, egg	1 oz.	23.0
Pancakes (from mix)	1 serving	8.0
Rolls		
Crescent	1	13.0
Frankfurter	1	20.0
Hamburger	1	20.0
Hard roll	1	30.0
Hoagie	1	72.0
Submarine	1	72.0
Breakfast cereals and other breakfast items		
Cereal		
Bran flakes	1 oz.	23.0
Corn flakes	1 oz.	24.0
Farina	1 cup	22.0
Granola	1 oz.	19.0
Oatmeal	1 cup cooked	27.0
Raisin bran	1 oz.	21.0

Foods	Amount	Grams of Carbohydrate
Corn muffin.............................	1 medium	20.0
Frozen waffle	1 serving	17.4
Pancakes (from mix)........................	1 serving	8.0

Chicken and poultry
Chicken
Fried, batter dipped breast with skin .	1	13.0
Drumstick with skin...........................	1	6.0
Fried, flour coated breast with skin ...	1	2.0
Drumstick with skin...........................	1	1.0
Roasted		
breast, no skin	1	0
Dark meat, no skin.........................	3 oz.	0
Drumstick with skin.......................	1	0
Drumstick, no skin.........................	1	0
Mixed meat with skin	3 oz.	0
Chicken hot dog...............................	1	3.0
Duck, roasted...............................	3 oz.	0
Goose, roasted	3 oz.	0
Turkey, roasted		
breast with skin	3 oz.	0
Dark meat with skin..........................	3 oz.	0
Leg with skin	3 oz.	0
Mixed meat with skin	3 oz.	0

Dairy Products
Butter and butter substitutes – see Fats and Oils
Cheese
American...	1 oz.	2.0
Camembert.......................................	1 oz.	0
Cheddar	1 oz.	0
Cottage		
Fat-free...	1 cup	10.0
Whole	1 cup	8.0
Cream cheese...................................	2 tbs.	1.0
Feta...	1 oz.	1.0
Mozzarella		
Part skim..	1 oz.	1.0
Whole milk......................................	1 oz.	1.0
Muenster..	1 oz.	1.0

Foods	Amount	Grams of Carbohydrate
Provolone	1 oz.	1.0
Ricotta		
Part skim milk	1 oz.	1.0
Whole milk	1 oz.	1.0
Romano	1 oz.	1.0
Swiss	1 oz.	1.0
Cream		
Heavy	1 Tbs.	0
Light	1 Tbs.	1.0
Sour	2 Tbs.	1.0
Eggs		
Fried	1	1.0
Hard boiled	1	1.0
Scrambled (milk & butter)	1	2.0
Half and half	1 Tbs.	1.0
Milk		
Low fat (1%)	8 fl. oz.	12.0
Low fat (2%)	8 fl. oz.	12.0
Skim	8 fl. oz.	12.0
Whole	8 fl. oz.	11.0
Plain yogurt		
Skim	1 cup	13.0
Whole	1 cup	12.0
Soy milk, unsweetened	1 cup	13.0
Desserts		
Breath mints	1	2.0
Brownie	1 serving	14.0
Cake		
Angel food	1 serving	30.0
Carrot	1 serving	35.0
Cheese, plain	1 serving	36.0
Chocolate	1 serving	38.0
Devil's food	1 serving	40.0
Pound	1 serving	19.0
Sheet cake with frosting	1 serving	77.0
White	1 serving	34.0
Yellow	1 serving	33.0
Cookies		
Chocolate chip	1 serving	7.0

Foods	Amount	Grams of Carbohydrate
Gingersnaps	1 serving	6.0
Peanut butter	1 serving	7.0
Sugar	1 serving	4.0
Vanilla wafers	1 serving	10.0
Ice cream		
Chocolate	¹/₂ cup	20.0
Vanilla	¹/₂ cup	15.0
Pie, homemade		
Apple	1 serving	60.0
Cherry	1 serving	60.0
Pumpkin	1 serving	37.0
Yogurt, frozen		
Chocolate	¹/₂ cup	24.0
Peach	¹/₂ cup	23.0
Vanilla	¹/₂ cup	23.0

Fats and Oils

Butter	1 Tbs.	0
Margarine	1 Tbs.	0
Mayonnaise	1 Tbs.	0
Mayonnaise substitute	1 Tbs.	0
Oil		
Canola	1 Tbs.	0
Corn	1 Tbs.	0
Olive	1 Tbs.	0
Peanut	1 Tbs.	0
Safflower	1 Tbs.	0
Soybean-cottonseed blend	1 Tbs.	0
Sunflower	1 Tbs.	0
Vegetable	1 Tbs.	0
Shortening, vegetable	1 Tbs.	0

Fish and shellfish

Abalone, canned	3 oz.	5.0
Bass, freshwater	3 oz.	0
Catfish, breaded	3 oz.	6.0
Cod	3 oz.	0
Crab	3 oz.	0
Eel	3 oz.	0
Grouper	3 oz.	0

Foods	Amount	Grams of Carbohydrate
Mussel	3 oz.	6.0
Lobster	3 oz.	0
Oyster		
Boiled or steamed	3 oz.	6.0
Breaded and fried	3 oz.	9.0
Salmon	3 oz.	0
Shark, batter dipped	3 oz.	5.0
Shrimp		
Boiled or steamed	3 oz.	0
Breaded and fried	3 oz.	9.0
Cocktail	4 oz.	19.0
Sushi	3 oz.	6.0
Trout	3 oz.	0
Tuna	3 oz.	0
Fruit		
Apple	1 medium	20.0
Applesauce, unsweetened	1 cup	28.0
Apricots	3 fresh	12.0
Avocado		
California	1	13.0
Florida	1	27.0
Banana	1	27.0
Blackberries	1 cup	18.0
Blueberries	1 cup	20.0
Cantaloupe	1/2 medium	22.0
Cherries	1 cup	20.0
Grapefruit, pink	1/2 medium	10.0
Grapes	10	9.0
Honeydew	1 cup	13.0
Kiwi	1 medium	9.0
Lemon	1	6.0
Lemon juice	1 Tbs.	1.0
Mango	1 cup	35.0
Orange	1 medium	16.0
Peach	1 (2 in.)	10.0
Pear	1 (3 in.)	21.0
Pineapple	1 cup	21.0
Plum	1 large	9.0
Prunes, dried (uncooked)	4 or 5	31.0

Foods	Amount	Grams of Carbohydrate
Raspberries	1 cup	14.0
Rhubarb (cooked with sugar)	1 cup	75.0
Strawberries	1 cup	12.0

Herbs

Allspice	1 tsp.	2.0
Basil	1 tsp.	1.0
Caraway	1 tsp.	1.0
Celery	1 tsp.	1.0
Cinnamon	1 tsp.	2.0
Coriander leaf	1 tsp.	0
Dill seed	1 tsp.	1.0
Garlic clove	1 clove	1.0
Ginger root (fresh)	1 oz.	4.0
Ginger root (ground)	1 tsp.	1.0
Saffron	1 tsp.	1.0
Thyme	1 tsp.	1.0
Vanilla (double strength)	1 tsp.	3.0

Legumes (cooked)

Black-eyed	1 cup	38.0
Lima	1 cup	34.0
Navy	1 cup	40.0
Red kidney	1 cup	40.0
Soybeans	1 cup	19.0
Split peas	1 cup	40.0
Tofu/bean curd	2 in. cube	3.0

Meats
Beef

Bottom round	3 oz.	0
Chuck	3 oz.	0
Ground beef	3 oz.	0
Rib	3 oz.	0
Steak		
Porterhouse	3 oz.	0
Sirloin	3 oz.	0
T-bone	3 oz.	0
Lamb	3 oz.	0
Pork		

Foods	Amount	Grams of Carbohydrate
Bacon	3 oz.	0
Canadian bacon	3 oz.	0
Ham	3 oz.	0
Veal	3 oz.	0
Venison	3 oz.	0
Nuts		
Almond paste	1 oz.	15.0
Almonds	1 oz.	6.0
Brazil	1 oz.	3.0
Cashews	1 oz.	8.0
Coconut	1 oz.	4.0
Hazelnuts (filberts)	1 oz.	5.0
Macadamia	1 oz.	5.0
Peanuts	1 oz.	4.0
Peanut butter	1 tbs.	3.0
Pecans	1 oz.	4.0
Pignolia	1 oz.	3.0
Pistachio	1 oz.	5.0
Pumpkin seeds	1 oz.	4.0
Sesame seeds	1 tbs.	1.0
Soybeans	¹/₂ cup	6.0
Sunflower seeds	1 oz.	6.0
Walnuts	1 oz.	4.0
Pasta and noodles		
Couscous	¹/₂ cup	20.0
Macaroni	¹/₂ cup	18.0
Noodles		
Chinese chow mein	¹/₂ cup	13.0
Egg	¹/₂ cup	19.0
Japanese somen	¹/₂ cup	25.0
Pasta		
Regular	¹/₂ cup	20.0
Spinach	¹/₂ cup	22.0
Whole wheat	¹/₂ cup	22.0
Pizza		
Cheese	1 slice	32.0

Foods	Amount	Grams of Carbohydrate
Cheese and pepperoni	1 slice	32.0
Vegetable	1 slice	30.0

Rice and rice dishes
Rice
Brown	¹/₂ cup	23.0
Pilaf	¹/₂ cup	21.0
White, instant	¹/₂ cup	20.0
White, long grain	¹/₂ cup	22.0
Wild rice	¹/₂ cup	18.0

Salads
Salad dressings
Blue cheese, regular	1 Tbs.	2.0
Caesar	1 Tbs.	1.0
Coleslaw dressing	1 Tbs.	3.0
Creamy Italian, low-calorie	1 Tbs.	2.0
French	1 Tbs.	2.0
Italian	1 Tbs.	0
Ranch	1 Tbs.	1.0
Russian	1 Tbs.	5.0
Thousand Island	1 Tbs.	2.0
Vinegar and oil	1 Tbs.	0
Salad toppings
Alfalfa sprouts	¹/₄ cup	0
Bacon bits	¹/₄ cup	8.0
Chinese noodles	¹/₄ cup	7.0
Croutons	¹/₄ cup	6.0
Taco chips	1 oz.	29.0
Vegetables – see Vegetables

Soups
Beef broth	1 cup	0
Beef with veg. and pasta	1 cup	16.0
Chicken consommé	1 cup	2.0
Chicken gumbo	1 cup	7.0
Clam chowder
Manhattan-style	1 cup	12.0
New England-style	1 cup	17.0
Cream of chicken	1 cup	15.0

Foods	Amount	Grams of Carbohydrate
Cream of mushroom	1 cup	15.0
French onion	1 cup	8.0
Minestrone	1 cup	16.0
Split pea with ham	1 cup	24.0
Tomato (made with milk)	1 cup	22.0
Turkey rice	1 cup	10.0
Vegetable	1 cup	16.0
Wonton	1 cup	8.0
Vegetables		
Asparagus	4 spears	3.0
Beans, green (boiled)	1/2 cup	5.0
Broccoli	1 cup	8.0
Brussels sprouts	1 cup	13.0
Cabbage	1 cup	4.0
Carrot	7 in.	7.0
Cauliflower	1 cup	5.0
Celery	1 stalk	1.0
Collards	1 cup	5.0
Corn	1 ear (5 in.)	16.0
Coleslaw	1 cup	9.0
Cucumber	1 cup	1.0
Dandelion greens	1 cup	7.0
Endive	1 cup	2.0
Kale	1 cup	7.0
Kohlrabi	1 cup	11.0
Lettuce		
Boston	1 cup	1.0
Iceberg	1 cup	2.0
Romaine	1 cup	2.0
Mushrooms	1 cup	3.0
Mustard greens	1 cup	5.0
Okra	1 cup	2.0
Onion	1 cup	12.0
Parsley	1 cup	1.0
Parsnips	1 cup	23.0
Peas, cooked	1 cup	11.0
Peppers		
Green (raw)	1 cup	4.0

Foods	Amount	Grams of Carbohydrate
Red (raw)	1 tsp.	4.0
Potato		
Baked (with skin)	1 medium	51.0
French fries		
Fried in oil	1 cup	28.0
Baked in oven	1 cup	24.0
Hash browns	1 cup	44.0
Mashed with milk	1 cup	25.0
Potato salad	1 cup	34.0
Pumpkin, canned	1 cup	20.0
Radish	10 large	3.0
Spinach, fresh	1 cup	2.0
Squash		
Summer	1 cup	8.0
Winter	1 cup	18.0
Sweet potato		
Baked	1 medium	37.0
Candied	1 cup	87.0
Tomato		
Canned	1 cup	10.0
Fresh	1 large	8.0
Juice	8 fl. oz.	10.0
Turnips		
Cooked	1 cup	8.0
Greens	1 cup	6.0
Yogurt		
Flavored	8 oz.	34.0
Plain, low-fat	8 oz.	16.0
Plain, nonfat	8 oz.	17.0
Plain, whole milk	8 oz.	11.0
With fruit	8 oz.	43.0
Yogurt, frozen		
Chocolate	¹/₂ cup	24.0
Peach	¹/₂ cup	23.0
Vanilla	¹/₂ cup	23.0

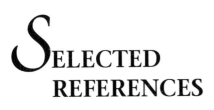

SELECTED REFERENCES

1. Acheson, KJ. Caffeine and coffee: their influence on metabolic rate and substrate utilization in normal weight and obese individuals. Am J Clin Nutr. 1980;33:989-997.

2. ACSM Position Stand on Exercise and Physical Activity for Older Adults. Med Sci. Sports. Exerc., Vol. 30, No. 6, pp.992-1008, 1998.

3. Adlercreutz H, Mazur W. Phyto-oestrogens and Western diseases. Ann Med 1997 Apr;29(2):95-120.

4. Ahuja JKC. Exler J, Raper N. 1997, Apr. 22. Data tables: Individual fatty acid intakes: results from 1995 continuing survey of food intakes by individuals.[Online]. ARS Food Surveys Research Group. Available (under "Releases") {visited 1998, April 22}.

5. Akinsola W, Smith F, Alimi T, Odewale F, Ladipo GO. Low protein/high calorie dietary regimen in the management of chronic renal failure. A preliminary study of Nigerian patients. Afr J Med Sci. 1991; Mar;20(1):53-9.

6. American College of Sports Medicine. Resource Manual for Guidelines for Exercise Testing and Prescription. Lea & Febiger. Philadelphia, PA, 1993.

7. American Heart Association. Why Should I Exercise? Pp. 18-19, 1994.

8. Anderson JJ, Metz JA. Contributions of dietary calcium and physical activity to primary prevention of osteoporosis in females. J Am Coll Nutr. 1993;12:378-383.

9. Anderson RA. Nutritional factors influencing the glucose/insulin system: chromium. J Am Coll Nutr. 1997;16(5):404-410.

10. Arthritis Foundation. Exercise and Your Arthritis. 1997.

11. Astrup A. Enhanced thermogenic responsiveness during chronic ephedrine treatment in man. Amer J Clin Nutr. 1985;42:83-94.

12. Astrup A, et al. The effect of ephedrine/caffeine mixture on energy expenditure and body composition in obese women. Metabolism: Clinical and Experimental. 1992 41;7:686-688.

13. Astrup A, Breum L, Tourro S, et al. The effect and safety of an ephedrine/caffeine compound compared to ephedrine, caffeine and placebo in obese subjects on an energy restricted diet. A double blind trial. International Journal of Obesity. 1991;15:359-366.

14. Ayehunie S. Inhibition of HIV-1 replication by an aqueous extract of Spirulina platensis (Arthrospira platensis). J Acquir Immune Defic Syndr Hum Retrovirol 1998; 18(1):7-12.

15. Balch, James F, M.D., and Balch, Phyllis A, C.N.C. Prescription for Nutritional Healing. New York: Avery Publishing Group Inc., 1990.

16. Batterman W. Whey protein for athletes. Dtsh Milchwirtsch. 1986;37(33):1010-1012.

17. Beal M, Matthews RT. Coenzyme Q10 in the central nervous system and its potential usefulness in the treatment of neurodegenerative diseases. Mol Aspects Med. 1997;18:s169-179.

18. Bellomo R. A prospective comparative study of moderate versus high protein intake for critically ill patients with acute renal failure. Renal Failure. 1997 Jan;19(1):111-20.

19. Berlin NI, Watkin DM, Gevirtz NR. Measurement of changes in gross body composition during controlled weight reduction in obesity by metabolic balance and body density-body water techniques. Metabolism 11:302, 1962.

20. Bernard S, Fouque C, Laville M, Zech P. Effects of low-protein diet supplemented with ketoacids on plasma lipids in adult chronic renal failure. Mineral Electrolyte Metabolism. 1996;22(1-3):143-6.

21. Bladt S, et al. Inhibition of MAO fractions and constituents of hypericum extract. J Geriatric Psychiatry Neurol. 1994;7(Supp 1):s57-59.

22. Block RJ, Weiss KW. Micro-Kjeldahl modification, in Amino Acid Handbook, Springfield, Ill., Charles C Thomas, 1956, p.11.

23. Borst S, Millard W, Lowenthal D. Growth hormone, exercise and aging: The future of therapy for the frail elderly. J Am Ger Soc 1994;42:528-535.

24. Bounous G. Immunoenhancing property of dietary whey protein in mice: role of glutathione. Clin Invest Med. 1989 Jun;12(3)154-161.

25. Bounous G. The biological activity of undenatured dietary whey protein: role of glutathione. Clin Invest Med. 1991;14(4):296-309.

26. Boza JJ. Nutritional value and antigenicity of two milk protein hydrolysates in rats and guinea pigs. J Nutr 1994;124(10):1978-1986.

27. Breum L, et al. Comparison of an ephedrine/caffeine combination and dexfenfluramine in the treatment of obesity. Int J Obesity. 1994;18:99-103.

28. British Nutrition Foundation. Unsaturated Fatty Acids: Nutritional and Physiological Significance. Chapman and Hall, London. 1992:152-163.

29. Britton HG. The chemical estimation of ketone bodies. Analyt. Biochem. 15:261, 1966.

30. Brochure: Folic Acid, The Vitamin that helps prevent birth defects; Distributed by the State of New York, Department of Health.

31. Bronner F. Nutrition and Health: Topics and Controversies. 1995 CRC Press, Boca Raton, FL.

32. Brocks A, Bandelow B, et. al. Aerobic exercise shown to relieve symptoms of panic disorder. American Journal of Psychiatry, Vol. 155, pp. 603-9, 1998.

33. Brouhard BH. The role of dietary protein in progressive renal disease. Am J Dis Child. 1986;Jul;140(7):630-7.

34. Bucci, L. Nutrients as Ergogenic Aids. CRC Press, Boca Raton, FL. 1994.

35. Burr ML, Fehily AM, Gilbert JF, et al. Effects of changes in fat, fish, and fibre intakes on death and myocardial reinfarction: diet and reinfarction trial (DART). Lancet 1989;2:757-62.

36. Cathcart EP. The influence of carbohydrates and fats on protein metabolism. J. Physiol. 39:311, 1999.

37. Chan JM, Stampfer MJ, et al. Plasma insulin-like growth factor-1 and prostate cancer risk: A prospective study. Science 1998;279(23):563-566.

38. Clark LC, Combs GF, Turnbull BW, Slate EH, Chalker DK, Chow J, Davis LS, Glover RA, Graham GF, Gross EG, Krongrad A, Lesher JL, Park HK, Sanders BB, Smith CL, Taylor JR. Effects of selenium supplementation for cancer prevention in patients with carcinoma of the skin: a randomized controlled trial. JAMA. 1996;276:1957-1963.

39. Clark, R. The somatogenic hormones and insulin like growth factor-1: Stimulators of lymphophoiesis and immune function. Endocrinal Rev 1997;137:1071-1079.

40. Cline GW, et. al. Impaired glucose transport as a cause of decreased insulin-stimulated muscle glycogen synthesis in type 2 diabetes. The New England Journal of Medicine. 1999;341;240-246.

41. Colgan, Michael, M.D. Optimum Sports Nutrition: Your Competitive Edge. Advanced Research Press. New York, NY, 1993.

42. Colker, CM., et al. Effects of citrus aurantium extract, caffeine and St. John's wort on body fat loss, lipid levels and mood states in overweight healthy adults. Current Therapeutic Research. 1999;60(3):145-153.

43. Colker CM, Kalman DS, Minsch A. Ephedra, caffeine and aspirin enhance fat loss under non exercising conditions. J Am Coll Nutr. 1997;16(5):501.

44. Colker CM, Torina GC, Swain MA, Kalman DS. Double-blind, placebo controlled evaluation of the safety and efficacy of ephedra, caffeine and salicin for short term weight reduction in overweight subjects. Journal of Exercise Physiology online. 1999;2(4):a26.

45. Connor WE. Omega-3 fatty acids and heart disease. In: Nutrition and Disease Update

Heart Disease. Eds. Kritchevsky D, Carroll KK, Champaign, IL. AOCS Press. 1994.

46. Connor WE, Connor SL. Omega-3 fatty acids from fish: primary and secondary prevention of cardiovascular disease. In: Bendich A, Deckelbaum R.eds. Preventive nutrition. Totowa, NJ: Humana Press, Inc. 1997:225-43.

47. Connor, WE, Should a low-fat high carbohydrate diet be recommended for every-one? The case for a low-fat high carb diet. N Eng J Med 1997;337:562-3, 566-7

48. Connor WE, Neuringer M, Reisbick S. Essential fatty acids: the importance of n-3 fatty acids in the retina and brain. Nutr Rev 1992;50:21-9.

48. Crestanello JA, Kamelgard J, Lingle DM, Mortensen SA, Rhode M, Whitman GJ. Elucidation of a tripartite mechanism underlying the improvement in cardiac tol-erance to ischemia by coenzyme Q10 pretreatment. J Thorac Cardiovascular Surg. 1996;111(2):443-450.

49. Cristofori FC, Duncan CG. Uric acid excretion in obese subjects during periods of total fasting. Metabolism 13:303, 1964.

50. Czeizel AE, Dudas I. Prevention of the first occurrence of neural tube defects by periconceptional vitamin supplementation. N Engl J Med. 1992;327:1832-1835.

51. Daly P, et al. Ephedrine, caffeine and aspirin: safety and efficacy for treatment of human obesity. Int J Obes Metab Disord. 1993;17: s73-78.

52. DeLeon D, Donovan S. Is breast cancer a potential side effect of GH treatment? Nature Medicine 1997;3(10):1081-1082.

53. DeLongeril M, Renaud S, Mamelle N, etal. Mediterranean alpha-linolenic acid-rich diet in secondary prevention of coronary heart disease. Lancet 1994;343:1454-9.

54. DiPietro L, Anda R, et al. Depressive symptoms and bodyweight. Int J Obesity 1993;17:485.

55. DiPierto L, Stunkard AJ, et al. Depressive symptoms and weight change in a national cohort of adults. Int J Obesity. 1992;16:745-753.

56. Dollemore, D. New Choices in Natural Healing. Rodale, Press, Inc., Emmaus, PA, 1995.

57. Dulloo AG. Ephedrine, xanthines and prostaglandin-inhibitors: actions and inter-actions in the stimulation of thermogenesis. Obesity. 1993;s17;1:s35-40.

58. Dulloo AG, et al. Potentiation of the thermogenic antiobesity effects of ephedrine by dietary methylxanthines: adenosine antagonism or phosphodiesterase inhibition. Metabolism: Clinical and Experimental 1992. 41;11:1233-1241.

59. Durnin J. Report of the IDECG Working Group on lower limits of energy and protein and upper limits of protein intakes. European Journal of Clinical Nutrition.1999;s174-s176.

60. Duyff, R. The ADA Complete Food and Nutrition Guide. Chronimed Publishing, Minneapolis, MN. 1996, pp. 85-86.

61. Ebben W, Jensen R. Strength Training for Women: debunking myths that block opportunity. The Physician and Sportsmedicine, Vol. 26, No. 5, pp. 86-97, 1998.

62. Elrick H. Exercise-the best prescription. The Physician and Sports medicine, Vol. 24, No. 2, p. 16ad, 1996.

63. Epstein FH, M.D., Shepherd PR, Ph.D., Kahn BB, M.D. Mechanisms of Disease. The New England Journal of Medicine. 1999;341;248-257.

64. FAO/WHO Expert Committee. Fats and Oils in Human Nutrition. Food and Nutrition Paper No. 57. FAO, Rome Italy. 1994.

65. Feinstein, A. Prevention's Healing With Vitamins. Rodale Press, Inc., Emmanus, PA., pp. 322-327, 1996.

66. Folkers K, Simonsen R. Two successful double-blind trials with coenzyme Q10 on muscular dystrophies and neurogenic atrophies. Biochem Biophys Acta. 1995;1271:281-286.

67. Foster S, Chongxi Y. Herbal Emissaries: Bringing Chinese Herbs to the West. Healing Arts Press, 1992. Rochester, VT.

68. Gamble JL. Physiological information from studies on the life raft ration. Harvey Lect. Ser. 42:247, 1946-47.

69. Garini G. Adherence to dietetic treatment, the nutritional metabolic status and the progression of chronic kidney failure. Ann Ital Med Int. 1992;April-June; 7(2):71-7.

70. Garlick P. Adaptation of protein metabolism in relation to high dietary protein intake. European Journal of Clinical Nutrition.1999;s34-s43.

71. Giese J. Proteins as ingredients: types, functions and applications. Food Technology 1994 Oct. 50-60.

72. Golan, Ralph, M.D. Optimal Wellness. 1995 Ballantine Books, NY.

73. Goodnight SH Jr, Harris WS, Connor WE, Illingwirth DR. Polyunsatuurated fatty acids, hyperlipidemia and thrombosis. Arteriosclerosis 1982;2:87-113.

74. Gretz N. Lasserre JJ, Hocker A, Strauch M. Effect of low-protein diet on renal function: are there definite conclusions from adult studies? Pediatr Nephrol. 1991;Jul;5(4):492-5.

75. Griffith, H. Winter, M.D. Complete Guide to Vitamins, Minerals & Supplements. Fisher Books. Tuscon, Az. 1988.

76. Grimsgaard S, Bonna K, Hansen JB, Nordoy A. Highly purified eicosapentaenoic acid and docosahexaenoic in humans have similar triacylglycerol lowering effect, but divergent effect on plasma lipoproteins and fatty acids. Am J Clin Nutr. 1997.

77. Harris, WS N-3 Fatty acids and serum lipoproteins: human studies. Am J Clin Nutr. 1997;65:1645S-1654S.

78. Haapakoski J, Malila N, Rautalahti M, Ripatti S, Maenpaa H, Teerenhovi L, Koss L,

Virolainen M, Edwards BK. Prostate cancer and supplementation with vitamin E in LDL oxidizability and prevention of atherosclerosis. Biofactors. 1998;7:51-54.

79. Hirai A, Terano T, Makuta H, Ozawa A, Fujita T, et al. Effect of oral administration of highly purified eicosapentaenoic acid and docosahexanenoic acid on platelet function and serum lipids in hyperlipideemic patients. Adv Prostag Thrombox Leuko Res. 1989;19:627-630.

80. Hu FB, Stampfer MJ, Manson JE, et al. Dietary intake of alpha linolenic acid and risk of fatal ischemic heart disease among women. Am J Clin Nutr 1999;69:890-7.

81. Hunt SM, Groff JL. Advanced Nutrition and Metabolism. West Publishing. 1990 St. Paul, MN.

82. Johnson RE, Passmore R, Sargent F. Multiple factors in experimental human ketosis. Arch. Intern. Med. 107:43, 1961.

83. Jones D, Gougeon R. Comparative double-blind study of Zhi-Thin™ and placebo as adjuncts to high-protein, low-calorie diets for weight loss. 1998 (Unpublished data) McGill University, Quebec, Canada.

84. Jung RT, Shetty PS. Caffeine: its effect on catecholamines and metabolism in lean and obese subjects. Clin Sci 1981;60:527-535.

85. Kang JX, Leaf A. Thee cardiac antiarrhythemic effects of polyunsaturated fatty acid. Lipids. 1996;31:S41-S44.

86. Katan MB. Should a low-fat high carbohydrate diet be recommended for everone? Beyond low fat diets. N Eng J Med 1997; 337:563-6.

87. Kang JX, Leaf A. Antiarrhythmic effects of polyunsaturated fatty acids: recent studies. Circulation 1996;94:1774-80.

88. Kekwick A, Pawan GLS. Calorie intake in relation to body weight changes in the obese. Lancet 2:155, 1956.

89. Kelly GS. Sports Nutrition: A Review of Selected Nutritional Supplements for Endurance Athletes. Alternative Medicine Review 1997; 2(4): 282-295.

90. Keville K. Herbs for Health and Healing. Emmaus, Pennsylvania: Rodale Press, Inc.;70, 105, 249.

91. Kinsella JE. Dietary fish oils: possible effect of n-3 polyunsaturated fatty acids in reduction of thrombosis and heart disease. Nutr Today. 1986:7-14.

92. Klatz R, Kahn C. Grow young with HgH: The amazing medically proven plan to reverse aging. 1997 Harper Collins, NY.

93. Kleinknecht C, Laouari D, Burtin M, Maniar S. Experimental approach to nutritional problems in chronic renal insufficiency. Annals of Pediatrics (Paris.) 1991;Jun;38(6):371-5.

94. Kris Etherton P. High monounsaturated fatty acid diets lower both plasma cholesterol and priacylglycerol concentrations.

95. Lamberts S, van den Beld A. The endocrinology of aging. Science 1997;278:419-424.

96. Leitamann M, Giovannucci E, Rimm E, Stampfer M, Spiege;lman D, Wing A, Willett W. The Relation of Physical Activity to Risk for Symptomatic Gallstone Disease in Men. Annals of Internal Medicine, Vol. 128, pp. 417-425, 1998.

97. Lemon PW. Is increases dietary protein necessary or beneficial for individuals with a physically active lifestyle? Nutrition Review. 1996;Apr 54(4 Pt 2):S169-75.

98. Lennox WC. Increase of uric acid in the blood during prolonged starvation. JAMA 82:602, 1924.

99. Lieberman, Shari, PhD, and Bruning, Nancy. The Real Vitamin & Mineral Book, 2ND ed. New York: Avery Publishing Group, 1997.

100. Linde K, et al. St John's Wort for depression: an overview and meta-analysis of randomized clinical trials. Brit Med Journal. 1996;313:253-258.

101. Macias WL, Alaka KJ, Murphy MH, Miller ME, Clark WR Mueller BA. Impact of the nutritional regimen on protein catabolism and nitrogen balance in patients with acute renal failure. J. of Par Ent Nut. 1996 Jan-Feb;20(1):56-62.

102. Mahan LK, Arlin M. Krause's Food, Nutrition and Diet Therapy. 8th edition. 1992. p 370. W.B. Saunders Company. Philadelphia, PA, 1992.

103. Mahan, L., Escott-Stump, S. Krause's Food, Nutrition and Diet Therapy 9th Edition. W.B. Saunders Company. Philadelphia, PA, 1996.

104. Marcus R, Butterfield G, et al. Effects of short term administration of recombinant growth hormone on elderly people. J Clin Endocrinal Metab 1990;70:519-527.

105. Matthew B. Evaluation of chemoprevention of oral cancer with Spirulina fusiformis. Nutr Cancer 1995; 24(2):197-202.

106. McArdle, W. Katch, F. Katch, V. Exercise Physiology Energy Nutrition and Human Performance. Lea & Febiger. Malvern, PA, 1991.

107. McLennan PL. Relative effects of dietary saturated, monounsaturated, and polyunsaturated fatty acids on cardiac arrhythmias in rats. Am J Clin Nutr. 1993;57:207-212.

108. Michaels GD, Margen S, Liebert G, Kinsell LW. Studies in fat metabolism. I. The colorimetric determination of ketone bodies in biological fluids. J. Clin. Invest. 20:1483, 1951.

109. Miller DK, Nation JR, Wellman PJ, Sensitization of anorexia and locomotion induced by chronic administration of ephedrine in rats. Life Science. 1999;65(5):501-511.

110. Mink B. Exercise and Chronic Obstructive Pulmonary Disease: modest fitness gains pay big dividends. The Physician and Sportsmedicine, Vol. 25, No. 11, pp. 43-52, 1997.

111. MRC Vitamin Study Research Group. Prevention of neural tube defects: results of the Medical Research Council vitamin study. Lancet. 1991;338:131-137.

112. Murray, Michael, N.D., Pizzorno, Joseph, N.D. Encyclopedia of Natural Medicine, 2nd ed. Prima Publishing. Rocklin, California. 1998.

113. Neuringer M, Connor WE. Lin DS, Barstad L, Luck S. Biochemical and functional effects of prenatal and postnatal omega-3 fatty acid deficiency on retina and brain in rhesus monkeys.ProcNatl Acad Sci USA 1986;83:4021-5.

114. Neuringer M, Connor WE, Van Petten C, Barstad L. Dietary omega-3 fatty acid deficiency and visual loss in infant rhesus monkeys. J Clin Invest 1984; 73:272-6.

115. Ng ST, Zhou J, et al. Growth hormone treatment induces mammary gland hyperplasia in aging primates. Nature Medicine 1997;3(10):1141-1144.

116. Nicolosi, RJ. Regulation of plasma lipoprotein levels by dietary triglycerides enriched with different fatty acids. Med Sci Sports Exerc 1997;29(11):1422-8.

117. Papadakis M, Grady D, Black D, et al. Growth hormone replacement in healthy older men improves body composition but not functional ability. Ann Intern Med 1996;124:708-716.

118. Pauls, Julie. Therapeutic Approaches to Women's Health. Aspen Publishers, Inc., 1995.

119. Peart, Brenda. Women Heart Health. 1997, Positive Promotions.

120. Pilkington TRE, Gainsborough H, Rosenoer VM, Carey M. Diet and weight-reduction in the obese. Lancet 1:856, 1960.

121. Position of The American Dietetic Association: vitamin and mineral supplementation. J Am Diet Assoc. 1996;96:73-77.

122. Pyka G, Lindenberger E. Muscle strength and fiber adaptations to a year long resistance training program in elderly men and women. J Gerontol 1994;49M22-27.

123. Rakosky J. Protein additives in foodservice applications. 1988. AVI, Van Nostrand Reinhold, New York.

124. Ramsey J. Energy expenditure, body composition, and glucose metabolism in lean and obese rhesus monkeys treated with ephedrine and caffeine. American Journal of Clinical Nutrition. 1998;68:42-51.

125. Reifenstein EC Jr., Albright F, Wells SL. The accumulation, interpretation, and presentation of data pertaining to metabolic balances, notably those of calcium, phosphorus, and nitrogen. J. Clin. Endocr. 5:367, 1945.

126. Renner E. Milk and dairy products in human nutrition. Munich, Germany, 1983.

127. Rimm EB, Willet WC, Hu FB, Sampson L, Colditz GA, Manson JE, Hennekens C, Stampfer MJ. Folate and vitamin B6 from diet and supplements in relation to risk

of coronary heart disease among women. JAMA. 1998;279:359-364.

128. Romay C. Antioxidant and anti-inflammatory properties of C-phycocyanin from blue-green algae. Inflamm Res, 1998;47(1):36-41.

129. Rudman D, Feller A. Effects of human growth hormone treatment in men over 60 years of age. New Eng J Med 1990;323:1-6.

130. Rudman D, Feller A, et al. Effects of human growth hormone on the body composition of elderly men. Horm Res 1991;36 (suppl 1):73-81.

131. Salahudeen AK, Hostetter TH, Raatz SK, Rosenberg ME. Effects of dietary protein in patients with chronic renal transplant rejection. Kidney Int. 1992;Jan;41(1):183-90.

132. Sastre J. Exhaustive physical exercise causes oxidation of glutathione status in blood: prevention by antioxidant administration. Am J Physiol. 1992;262 (5pt2):R992-995.

133. Schapp GH, Bilo HJ, van der Meulen J, Oe PL, Donker AJ. Effect of changes in daily protein intake on renal function in chronic renal insufficiency: differences in reaction according to disease entity Nephron. 1993;63(2):207-15.

134. Schumm DE. Essentials of Biochemistry. Second Edition, p 325. 1995 Little, Brown and Company, New York.

135. Shaffer, PA. Antiketogenesis. IV. The ketogenic-antiketogenic balance in man and its significance in diabetes. J. Biol. Chem. 54:399, 1922.

136. Shils ME, Olson JA, Shike M, Ross AC: Modern Nutrition in Health and Disease, 9th ed. Baltimore: Williams & Wilkins, 1999, pp.647-8, 1409.

137. Silica Hydride Web Site: abkit@msn.com ultimate.html

138. Simopoulos AP. Genetics and nutrition: or what your genes can tell you about nutrition. In: Simopoulos AP, Childs B,eds. Genetic variation and nutrition. World Rev Diet. 1990;63:25-34.

139. Simopoulos AP. Omega-3 fatty acids in health and disease and in growth and development. Am J Clin Nutri. 1991;54:438-63.

140. Siscovick DS, Raghunathan TE, King I, et al. Dietary intake and cell membrane levels of long-chain n-3 polyunsaturated fatty acids and the risk of primary cardiac arrest. JAMA 1995;274:1364-7.

141. Soybeans; Healthcare Guide. United Soybean Board 1997 St. Louis, MO.

142. Strom H, et al. Comparison of a carbohydrate rich diet and diets rich in stearic or palmitic acid in NIDDM patients. Diabetes Care 1997;20(12):1807.

143. Stryer L: Biochemistry, 4rth ed. New York: W.H. Freeman and Company, 1995, pp. 770-1.

144. Surgeon General's Report on Physical Activity and Health. Cancer Facts and Figures. American Cancer Society, 1997.

145. Taaffe D, Jin I. Lack of effect of recombinant human growth hormone (GH) on muscle morphology and GH-insulin like growth factor expression in resistance trained elderly men. J Clin Endocrinol Metab 1996;81:421-425.

146. The 1st Annual Conference on the Therapeutic Applications of Coenzyme Q10. 1997.

147. The Burton Goldberg Group. Alternative Medicine - The Definitive Guide.

148. Future Medicine Publishing, Inc. Puyallup, Washington. 1993.

149. Thiede HM. Inhibition of MAO and COMT by hypericum extracts and hypericin. J Geriatric Psychiatry Neurol 1994;7 (Supp 1):s54-56.

150. Tyler VE. Herbs of Choice: The Therapeutic Use of Phytomedicinals. 1994, Pharmaceutical Products Press New York.

151. US Department of Agriculture, Agricultural Research Service. 1998.

152. USDA Nutrient Database for Standard Reference, Release 12. Nutrient Data Laboratory.

153. Vergal RG, Sanchez BL, Heredero BL, Rodriguez PL, Martinez AJ. Primary prevention of neural tube defects with folic acid supplementation: a Cuban experience. Prenat Diagn. 1990;10:149-152.

154. Vorbach EU, et al. Effectiveness and tolerance of the hypericum extract LI 160 in comparison to imipramine: randomized double blind study with 135 outpatients. J Getriatr Psychiatry Neurol 1994; 7(Supp 1):s19-24. W.B. Saunders Company, Philadelphia, PA. 1996, pp. 106-108.

155. Webber PC. Fischer S, VonSchacky C, et al. Dietary omega-3 polyunsaturated fatty acids and eicosanoid formation in man. In: Simopoulos, Kifer RR, Martin RE(eds) Health Effects of Polyunsaturated Fatty Acids in Seafood's. Orlando, Academic Press, 1976:49-60.

156. White F, Shannon JS, Patterson RE. Relationship between vitamin and calcium supplement use and colon cancer. Cancer Epidemiol Biomarkers Prec. 1997;6:769-774.

157. Whitney, E., Cataldo, C., Rolfes, S. Understanding Normal and Clinical Nutrition. West Publishing, Minneapolis, MI., pp. 667-686, 1994.

158. Whitney E, Hamilton E, Rolfes S. Understanding Nutrition. Fifth Edition. 1990 West Publishing, St. Paul, MN.

159. Wolinsky, I. Nutrition in Exercise and Sport, Third Edition. 1998. CRC Press, Boca Raton, Fl.

160. Worthington BS, Taylor LE. Balanced low-calorie vs. high-protein-low-carbohydrate reducing diets. Journal of the American Dietetic Association. 1974;Jan 64(1):47-51.

$\mathcal{I}$NDEX

Dr. Colker's recommendations are his own. He does not make money from, or profit in any way by, the sale of products mentioned or recommended in this book.

To make a personal appointment with Dr. Colker, or any of the Greenwich Diet physicians, dietitians, exercise physiologists, or clinical counselors, write or email *Peak Wellness, Inc.* at:

Peak Wellness, Inc.
50 Holly Hill Lane
Greenwich, CT 06830
www.peakwell@idt.com